"THE MOST REVOLUTIONARY ADVANCE"

When *Sports Illustrated* finally publicized "the most revolutionary advance in athletic training methods in recent years," the Isometric Era began.

Now this scientific breakthrough can be harnessed not just by champion athletes, but in a general program of physical fitness for boys and girls and men and women of all ages.

Henry Wittenberg has often demonstrated in person and on television the magic of isometrics which he used in his own Olympic championship careei, and which he now uses as a college coach.

ISOMETRICS, unique among physical fitness manuals, embodies "all the scientific principles that govern physical improvement in the shortest possible time."

So whether your goal is reducing, firming or strengthening your body or any portion of it, here is the newest and most reliable plan for you. It is a plan that you can start in *seconds a day* in your own home, or even while at work, without any equipment, and in perfect safety.

ABOUT THE AUTHOR

HENRY WITTENBERG has had a long and successful career in athletics and physical education. He holds a B.S. degree from C.C.N.Y. and a Masters degree in physical education from Columbia University.

As an amateur wrestler, he compiled the most impressive record in that sport in U.S. history, and is considered by experts to be the greatest wrestler of all time. From 1940 to 1952 he wrestled in the 191-pound and heavyweight divisions in this country and abroad, and remained undefeated after more than 400 consecutive matches! During this time, he was eight times National A.A.U. champion. He won the coveted Gold Medal for wrestling at the 1948 Olympic Games in London.

Since his retirement from active competition in 1953, Wittenberg has devoted his time to teaching. He has coached the New York City Police Department team, and in 1959 was named the U.S. National Coach for the American wrestling tour to Russia, Turkey, Bulgaria and Poland. He is a member of the U.S. Olympic Committee and the National Amateur Athletic Union Wrestling Committee. At present he coaches wrestling and teaches physical education at Yeshiva University in New York.

The theory of isometric contractions is not new to Wittenberg. He had read how the legendary wrestler Farmer Burns practiced his scissors grip by placing a sack of grain between his legs and squeezing it until it burst. Experimenting further, Wittenberg practiced holds on a football dummy, exerting *pressure without motion.* This contributed much to his success on the mat, but it was not until a few years ago, when the principles of isometric contraction became generally regarded as a breakthrough in the field of physical fitness, that he completed his experiments.

Based on research with students, businessmen and athletes, Wittenberg has now compiled this manual, which embodies all the scientific principles that govern physical improvement in the shortest possible time.

ISOMETRICS

THE AMAZING NEW 10-SECOND
SYSTEM OF NO-MOTION EXERCISES FOR
FIGURE CONTROL, STRENGTH AND HEALTH
ILLUSTRATED WITH OVER 150 PHOTOS

by HENRY WITTENBERG

Fully Illustrated

AWARD BOOKS
NEW YORK

TANDEM BOOKS
LONDON

SEVENTH AWARD PRINTING 1970

AWARD BOOKS are published by
Universal Publishing and Distributing Corporation
235 East Forty-fifth Street, New York, N. Y. 10017

TANDEM BOOKS are published by
Universal-Tandem Publishing Company Limited
14 Gloucester Road, London SW7, England

Manufactured in the United States of America

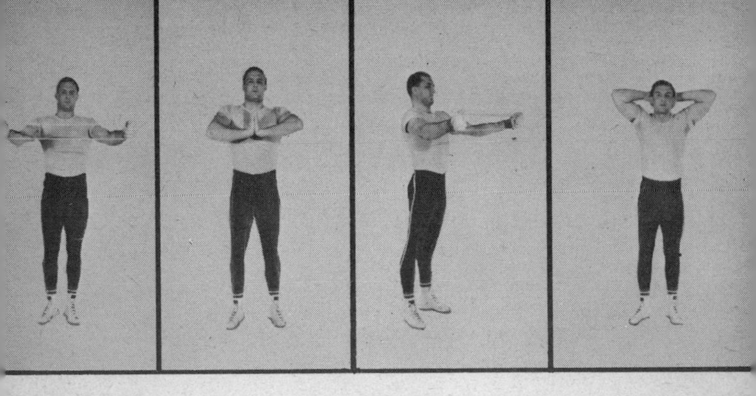

CONTENTS

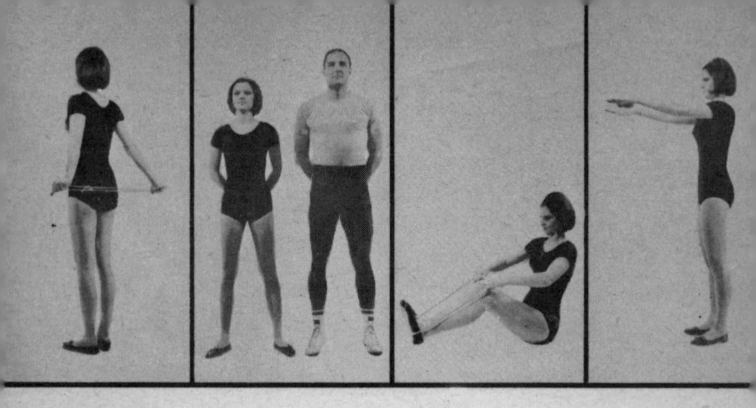

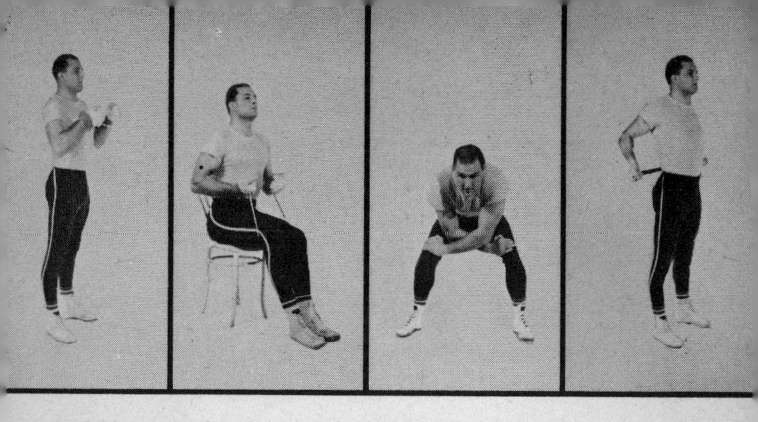

PART III

The champions of tomorrow can be found in the ranks of the young people who are building their bodies today. Physical fitness is the foundation for all sports—and their real purpose.

In or out of competition, physical fitness is also the basis of a nation's health and well-being. Physical fitness programs are most effective when they are begun at an early age and maintained throughout the active lifetime of every citizen.

—Arthur G. Lentz
Asst. Executive Director
U.S. Olympic Committee

FOREWORD

The simplicity of the exercises in this plan makes it ideally suited to the needs of people of all ages and both sexes who wish to follow the physical-fitness path to vitality and happiness. Isometric exercises are self-regulating, and have built-in limits. Since your own muscles determine the counter-force, there is no danger as there would be in lifting too heavy a weight, etc.

Any exercise in this book may be attempted by a female exerciser, from teen-age girl to middle-age woman, or by a male exerciser from boy to older man. Just remember to follow the instructions at the start of each section and exercise, and not to skip levels.

It is assumed that women will be more interested in their section, which is devoted to slimming and firming, than in the men's section, which emphasizes increase in musculature and strength. But the entire program is useful and safe for everyone.

But even the magic of isometrics-isotonics should begin with a word of reminder.

A medical checkup should precede any exercise plan for any individual. (People with special physical problems, especially, should never start any physical-fitness program without checking with their doctors.) Besides supplying you with valuable information about your present condition, the checkup might very well indicate that you can freely proceed to a higher level in this program than you thought possible.

The author and publishers of this book are certain that the exercises in this plan will do just what they promise to. Readers must study the text carefully before starting, paying special attention to the author's well-founded suggestion: **Do not skip levels.** Proceed from one to the next in the sequence indicated.

You will find many other similar training tips along the way.

In exercise, as in many other things, moderation is still the best rule.

ISOMETRICS

Dedicated to
the devoted and tireless workers
of the Amateur Athletic Union
of the United States whose efforts
on behalf of youth
ensure a more fit and
healthier America.

PART I

SO YOU WANT TO GET IN SHAPE . . .

If you have been feeling that you should do something about improving your physical condition, you couldn't have picked a better time than this to start. For now physiologists have discovered that total physical fitness can be achieved amazingly fast and without special equipment.

The value of regular exercise is also psychological, for as physical condition improves, the capacity to enjoy all phases of living is heightened.

Some of the obstacles preventing many people from achieving fitness are the relative lack of physical activity in daily living, and the scarcity of time available for a regular exercise program. We are always too busy, and getting to a gym can be time consuming. Thus "weekend athletes," in their enthusiasm, often do themselves more harm than good. Unfortunately, the less one does, the less one feels like doing, and the body's aging processes take over.

In the 1920s, an interesting phenomenon was observed by scientists studying the effects of inactivity upon muscles. In an experiment, the legs of frogs were bound together to prevent movement, and kept that way for relatively long periods. Surprisingly, when the bindings were removed the leg muscles of the tied frogs were larger and stronger than those of a control group whose legs were left untied. What had happened? The frogs that had had their legs tied strained continually throughout the test period, and the effect of contracting and tensing their muscles against the bonds resulted in remarkable development.

This form of static exercise is used by physiotherapists in the field of physical rehabilitation, with valuable results particularly in patients required to wear casts for long periods. But it remained for two German physiologists, Hettinger and Muller, in 1953, to apply this technique to healthy individuals and to scientifically measure the results. Their research revealed that the intense contraction of a muscle against a fixed object increased strength as much as 5% in *one week* although a complete exercise was done for only *6 seconds,* and only once a day. Subsequent findings by dozens of other researchers supported this conclusion. One doctor reported strength increases up to 300%! Today, this discovery is being put to practical use by athletes and coaches around the world.

In 1961, Dr. Jay Bender of Southern Illinois University led the Pennant-winning Pittsburgh Pirates through an amazingly successful program of this new technique.

Olympic weightlifters Lou Riecke and Bill March broke their own records by training with this method. Their coach, Bob Hoffman, the dean of body builders, believes this technique to be the most remarkable breakthrough in the entire area of physical fitness.

From basketball players to swimmers, athletes have incorporated this new way to increase strength into their training programs. Almost no athlete would omit a daily session of this technique in his routine. As records continue to be broken by trainees using this method, its effectiveness is evident.

This new concept in building strength and muscles is known as *Isometric Contraction.*

WHAT IS AN ISOMETRIC CONTRACTION?

An *isometric* contraction is the action of a muscle or group of muscles against an immovable object, or against each other, creating *tension without motion.* The expression "lifting oneself up by the bootstraps" is an accurate description of an *isometric* exercise.

To perform a typical isometric contraction, place your

right hand against the right side of your head. Now *push your hand against your head* and *at the same time push back with your head.* Equalize the pressure so that both head and hand are pushing against each other with precisely the same force and there is a *motionless* deadlock.

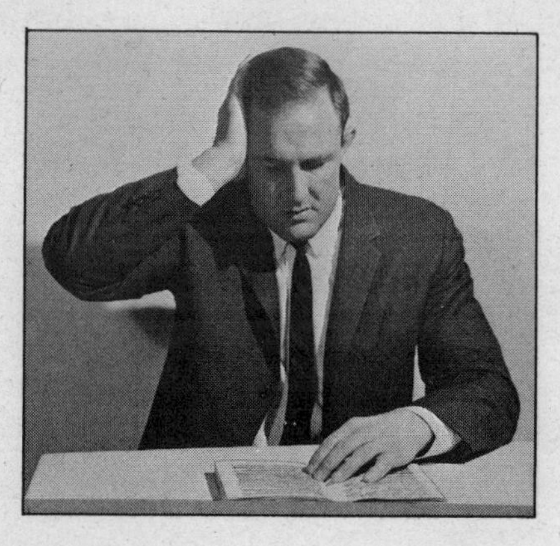

As you do this, lightly press the fingertips of your left hand to the right side of your neck. Notice how firm the muscles become as you increase the tension. Now relax. You have completed an isometric contraction. The muscles that contracted were working in direct proportion to the amount of strain that you voluntarily exerted upon them. In this form of effort, more muscle fibers are contracted at one time than in any other type of exercise.

As you push more strenuously against an immovable object, oxygen within the muscle fibers is rapidly burned and calories are consumed. The muscle in its contracted state also expands, and this expansion, by constricting the blood vessels, prevents fresh oxygen from coming to the muscle. As you increase tension, you inevitably reach *maximum effort,* the point at which pressure can no longer be increased.* You are also applying the *overload*

* The point of maximum effort is demonstrated when: 1. You cannot increase the force of the contraction. 2. The muscles involved involuntarily quiver from the tension applied.

principle to the muscles involved. This overloading causes the *oxygen deficit phenomenon,* a condition where the shortage of oxygen to the muscles affected quickly produces acute fatigue.

In all isometric exercises, it is essential to reach the overload stage to insure maximum benefits, because the body reacts to this effect by rebuilding the muscles involved to a much greater extent than they were before the contraction. Tendons and ligaments are also positively affected, resulting in added strength, posture improvement, body tone and a better general appearance.

ISOTONIC OR PHASIC EXERCISES

Until recently, the only type of exercise used in fitness programs was the *isotonic* or phasic. This is exercise *with movement:* throwing a ball or walking, for instance. Isotonic exercises tend to become time-consuming and tedious: the more one does them, the more they must be repeated to be of value. In order to maintain a high level of fitness employing this type of exercise, one would have to work out several hours a day. The inclusion of *isometrics* in a workout, however, gives better results—and in a fraction of the time.

The value of selected *isotonic* exercises in a total fitness program is demonstrated in two areas:

First: The preliminary warm-up period. Physical exertion requires physical preparation. You should prepare for the increase in bodily effort by warming up. A few simple stretching and bending movements are necessary to avoid muscle and ligament strain.

Second: Cardiovascular conditioning. Isotonic exercises are effective in the development and improvement of the heart and circulatory system. The massaging and kneading action of moving muscles upon the blood vessels, plus the necessity for the heart to send blood to working areas of the body, are essential to the proper functioning and health of these organs.

Thus, the benefits of incorporating both isotonics and isometrics in a total-fitness program are apparent. The results include: increased cardiovascular efficiency and endurance; increased body strength and vigor; improvement of muscle tone and contour.

HOW FAR DO YOU WISH TO GO?

Before answering this question, consider some practical factors. Age is important in determining the extent to which you should develop your level of fitness, using *any* fitness plan. The program that follows is designed to offer a *gradual* increase in efficiency and power. As your capacity to exercise improves, you will move from one level to the next without strain. Those over 40 may wish to remain at an earlier, less demanding level for a longer period of time. Some may simply wish to exercise just enough to improve general well-being. Others may wish to use the program to improve performance in competitive sports.

Regardless of the basis for starting an isometric-isotonic fitness program, it is essential that the exercises be done *every day*. Naturally, if you spend an afternoon shovelling snow or playing several sets of tennis, you may eliminate that day's workout period. But, except for illness, there should be no other reason for skipping a workout in any one day.

Whenever you are unable to hold your regular *isometric-isotonic* workout period, you should then substitute the *alternate isometric* period. This takes less than two minutes to complete and can be done anywhere. This alternate period is basic to the total fitness plan: if this alone is done, daily, there will still be a substantial increase in strength and a tightening-up of flabby muscles.

Since isometric contractions permit you to put only as much effort into an exercise as you, as an individual, can, the danger of harming yourself is reduced to a minimum. This aspect of individual ability makes isometrics an ideal form of exercise for women.

It is advisable, however, that you consult with your doctor and have a checkup before starting this or any other fitness plan. You may discover that you are not in as good physical condition as you think you are. On the other hand, the checkup may indicate a much higher physical-fitness goal for you than seemed possible.

Everyone entering the isometric-isotonic fitness plan *must* start at the Primary Level, regardless of age or physical condition. Since this is a new way to exercise, it will call on all your resources, no matter how good your condition at the start. You will obtain maximum benefits from the outset, and after a few days of working out in the plan, you should experience a new, exhilarating feeling of well-being.

Do not rush the program or skip levels.

As total fitness improves through the Primary Level, you may continue to the Secondary Level, although people over 40 may wish to remain at the Primary for the reasons mentioned before. Thus, unusually vigorous persons of that age level, or those wishing to participate in sports, will want to proceed to the Secondary which is supplemented by isometric contractions as applied to particular sports.

Level three, or Peak Level, is designed for adults under the age of 40 who have progressed through the first two Levels and wish to achieve a high degree of physical efficiency. It is also useful to athletes during off-season periods, or as a substitute workout when they cannot participate in their regular training programs.

FITNESS AND BODY WEIGHT

If you are over 25 years of age and have gained ten pounds over the past year, chances are that you have been averaging an intake of 100 excess calories a day. The exercises in this program, at each level, are designed to burn away at least that amount of calories per workout. An intake of 100 fewer calories a day *plus* the workout will cause a corresponding drop in weight.

As your fitness level increases more calories will be burned. By regulating your caloric intake, then, you can reach the weight level you desire. Should you wish to maintain your present weight as your workout level rises, simply eat more. Since you will be turning fat to muscle, and since muscle is firmer than fat, you will actually be slimmer, more trim, though your weight remains the same. Basic body type, however, is an inherited characteristic. If, for example, you are naturally stocky, no amount or type of exercise can make you long and rangy. What exercise *can* do for you is give you a trimmer, stronger, better-functioning physique.

As your physical condition improves, through the following course of *total* fitness, your appetite will also increase. This is in keeping with over-all physical improvement. But only you can control your desire to eat in relation to the weight you wish to maintain. Diet should be tempered with reason as you train. A combination of exercise and diet is the best way to keep at your optimum weight while maintaining a high level of physical vigor. The four major food divisions are Meat, including Fish and Eggs, Dairy Products, Vegetables, and Grains. You should eat at least one food from each of these divisions daily.

PART II

THE ISOMETRIC-ISOTONIC TOTAL-FITNESS PLAN

This *plan* is divided into three levels:

★ Primary Level
★ ★ Secondary Level
★ ★ ★ Peak Level

Each *level* is divided into three periods:

Warm-up Period
Isometric Period
Isotonic Period

These periods are interrelated and should be done in the sequence described. Nothing should be omitted. Carefully read the instructions preceding each exercise period, particularly with reference to the isometrics. The common element in *all* the exercises is the use of *time.*

The duration of each exercise is indicated. In the case of the *isometric* contractions, it remains constant: 10 seconds. The time element changes in the *isotonic* exercises as physical condition improves. *Keep within the time limit of your particular level.* The total time for any daily workout will never exceed 12 minutes.

The plan also includes an alternate isometric period which is to be used when it is impractical to go through the three periods called for in the daily workout. It will allow you to maintain your level of efficiency without backsliding.

★ PRIMARY LEVEL

The primary level is indicated for those starting the Isometric-Isotonic Plan for the first time. The exercises described in this section will materially increase your strength regardless of your physical condition at the outset. Adequate total physical fitness can be reached and maintained at this level.

The total time for the primary level workout is at least 10 but never more than 12 minutes a day.

The following charts should be followed to measure your rate of improvement, for, as your fitness improves you will be required to do more repetitions at greater speeds. This applies **ONLY** to the **isotonic** period. The warm-up period always remains the same. While the **isometric** period also remains the same, the amount of work will automatically increase as strength increases.

★ PRIMARY LEVEL

CHART I

First and Second Weeks

Follow this chart every day for *two weeks*

	Exercise	*Repetitions*	*Time in Secs*
WARM-UP	1. Bend and Stretch	12	30
	2. Squat and Touch	10	30
	3. Knee Hug	10	30
	4. Twist and Touch	10	45
	5. Seal Bend	10	40
ISOMETRIC	1. Parade Rest	1	10
	2. Palm Push	1	10
	3. Two-Hand Curl	1	10
	4 Front Cable Stretch	1	10
	5. Neck Press	1	10
	6. Hip Press	1	10
	7. Overhead Cable Stretch	1	10
	8. Triceps Push	1	10
	9. Back Cable Stretch	1	10
	10. Dead Lift	1	10
ISOTONIC	1. Jumping Jack	12	15
	2. Front Waist Bend	12	30
	3. Squat Thrust	10	30
	4. Knee Push-ups	10	25
	5. Imaginary Rope Skip	60	30

CHART II

Third Week – Follow this chart every day for *one week*

	Exercise	*Repetitions*	*Time in Secs*
WARM-UP	1. Bend and Stretch	12	30
	2. Squat and Touch	10	30
	3. Knee Hug	10	30
	4. Twist and Touch	10	45
	5. Seal Bend	10	40
ISOMETRIC	1. Parade Rest	1	10
	2. Palm Push	1	10
	3. Two-Hand Curl	1	10
	4. Front Cable Stretch	1	10
	5. Neck Press	1	10
	6. Hip Press	1	10
	7. Overhead Cable Stretch	1	10
	8. Triceps Push	1	10
	9. Back Cable Stretch	1	10
	10. Dead Lift	1	10
ISOTONIC	1. Jumping Jack	24	30
	2. Front Waist Bend	15	30
	3. Squat Thrust	12	30
	4. Knee Push-ups	14	30
	5. Imaginary Rope Skip	90	45

★ PRIMARY LEVEL

WARM-UP PERIOD

The following five exercises are designed to prepare you for the more strenuous activity that comes later. These should always be done before starting on the isometric or isotonic periods. Keep within the time limit indicated for each exercise. Do not increase the number of repetitions. Proceed immediately from one exercise to the next. At the completion of the warm-up period, your heart, musculature and blood stream will be prepared to handle the added effort needed to do the subsequent exercises. These exercises will stimulate, not tire you.

Total time for this period: 3 minutes. Keep a stop-watch or a clock with a sweep-second hand within view so that you can time each exercise.

BEND AND STRETCH

This exercise should be repeated *12 times.*

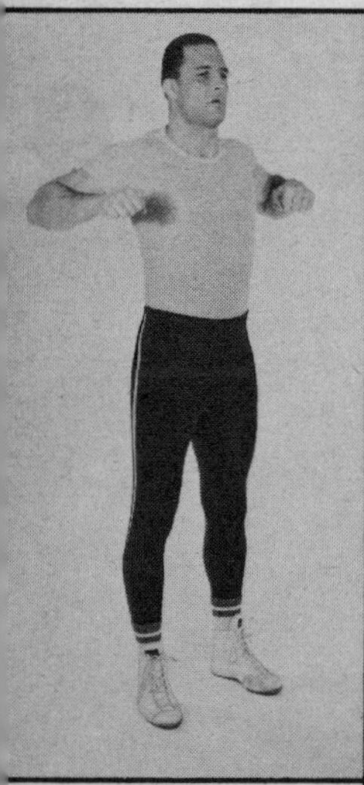

Start position: Stand erect, arms at shoulder level, fists clenched, elbows bent and thrust back as far as possible.

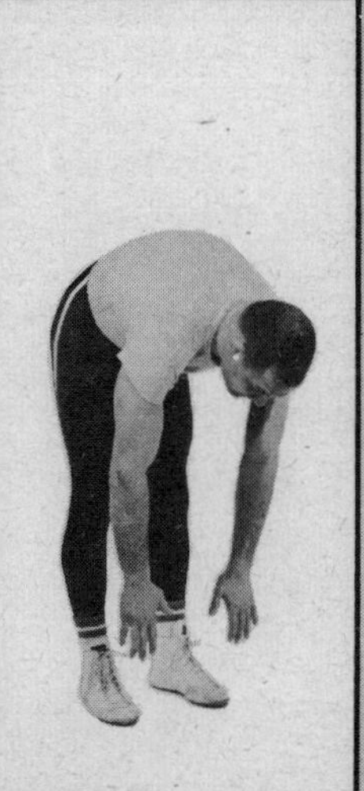

Action-Count 1. Bend forward to floor, with arms hanging down and fingers relaxed. Bend knees slightly and allow head to hang forward.

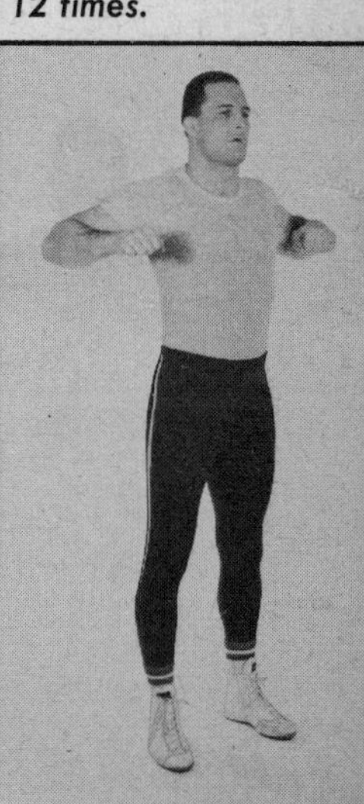

Count 2. Return to start position.

★ **PRIMARY LEVEL**
Warm-up #2
Time: 30 seconds

SQUAT AND TOUCH

This exercise should be repeated *10 times.*

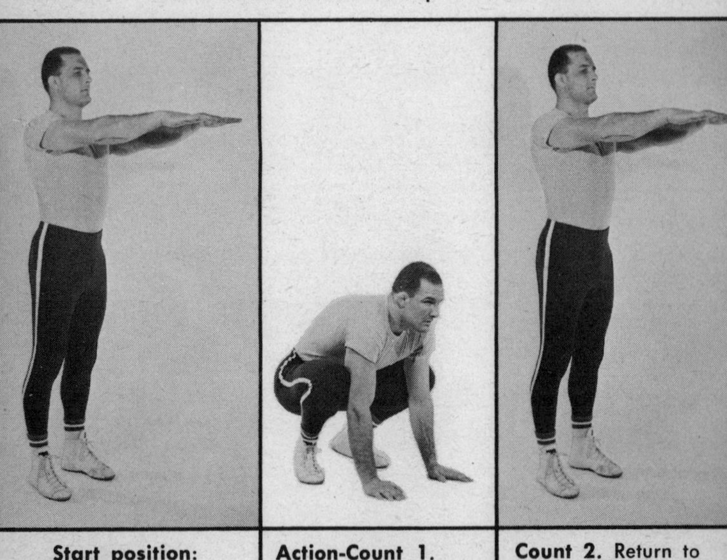

Start position: Stand erect, arms extended to front, palms down, feet about 12 inches apart.

Action-Count 1. Bend knees and squat, touching fingers or palms of hands to floor between knees. Keep head erect and back straight.

Count 2. Return to start position.

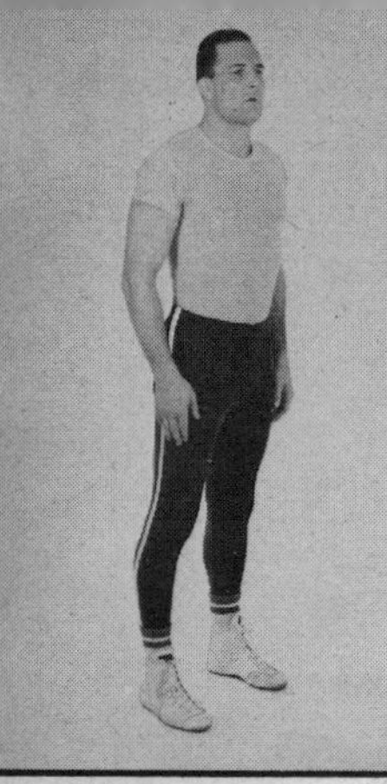

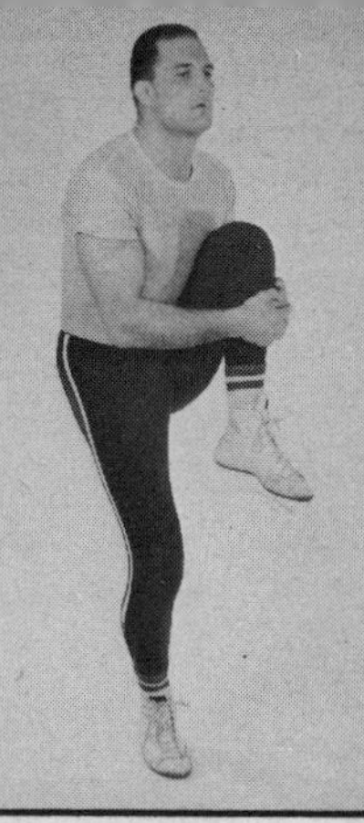

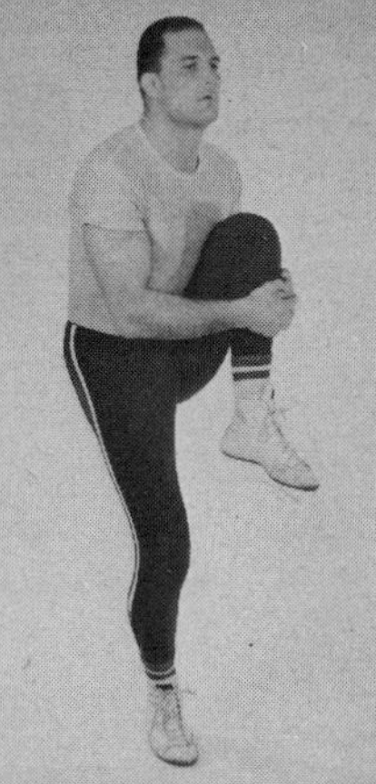

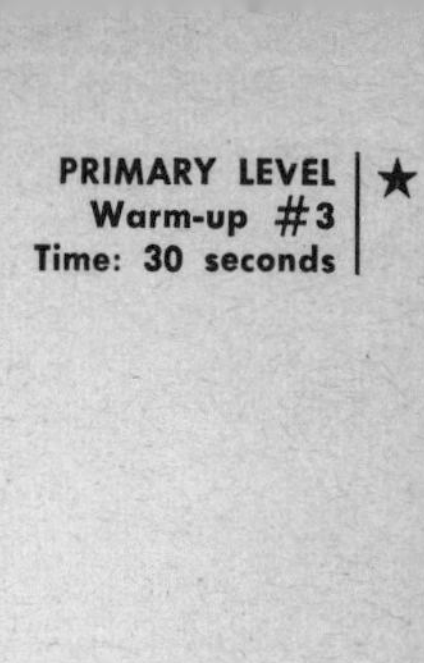

PRIMARY LEVEL ★
Warm-up #3
Time: 30 seconds

Start position: Stand erect, back straight, arms at sides.

Action-Count 1. Raise left knee to chest level. Grasp lower leg with both arms and draw leg to chest. Keep back straight.

KNEE-HUG

This exercise should be repeated *10 times,* and each repetition represents 4 counts.

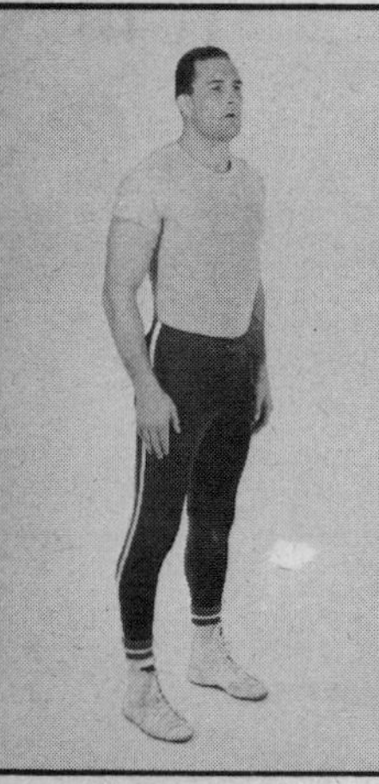

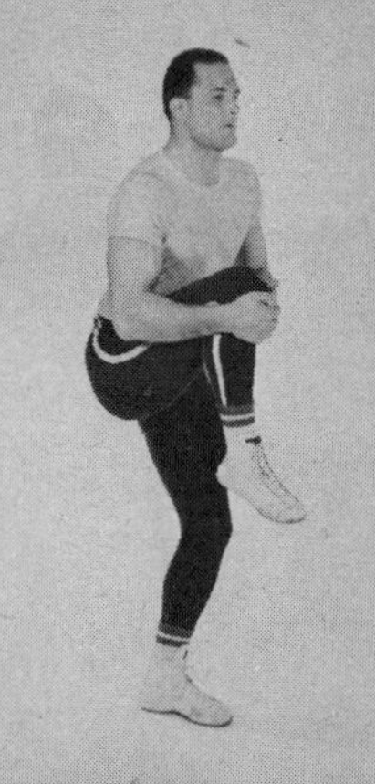

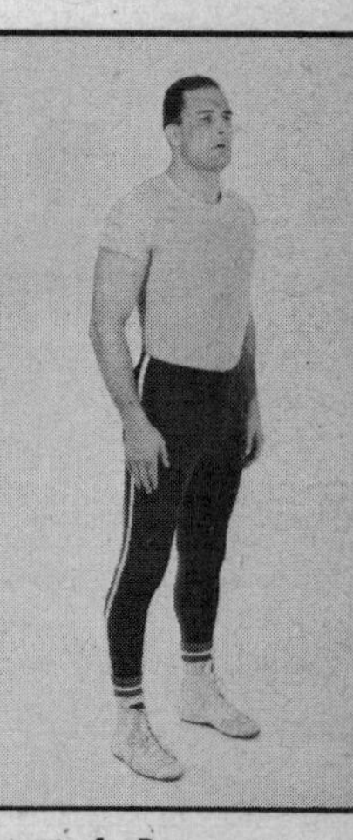

Count 2. Return to start position.

Count 3. Raise right knee to chest as in Count 1.

Count 4. Return to start position.

★ **PRIMARY LEVEL**
Warm-up #4
Time: 45 seconds

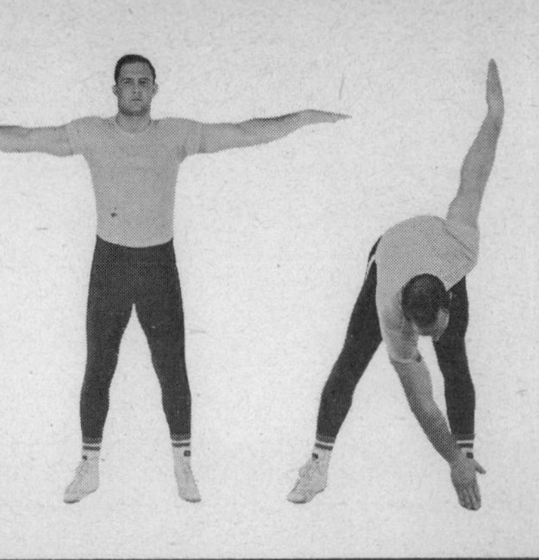

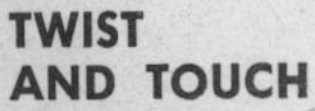

TWIST AND TOUCH

This exercise should be repeated *10 times*, and each repetition represents 4 counts.

Start position: Stand erect, arms extended at sides, palms down, legs apart.

Action-Count 1. Twist to left, touching right fingertips to left toe, extending left arm vertically. (Left knee may be slightly bent.)

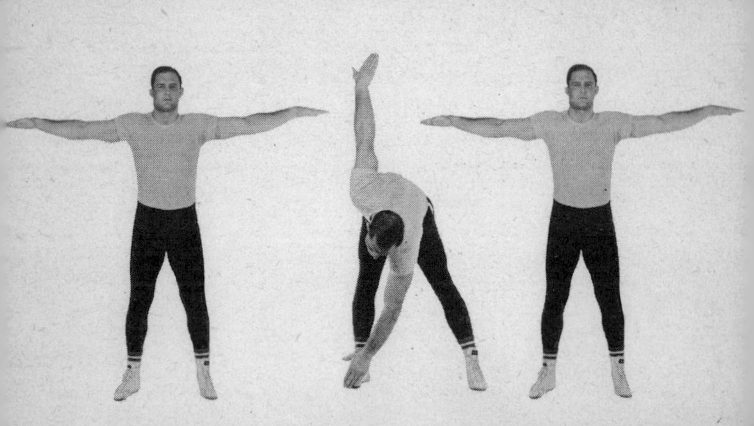

Count 2. Return to start position.

Count 3. Repeat Action-Count 1, but in opposite direction.

Count 4. Return to start position.

SEAL BEND

This exercise should be repeated *10 times.*

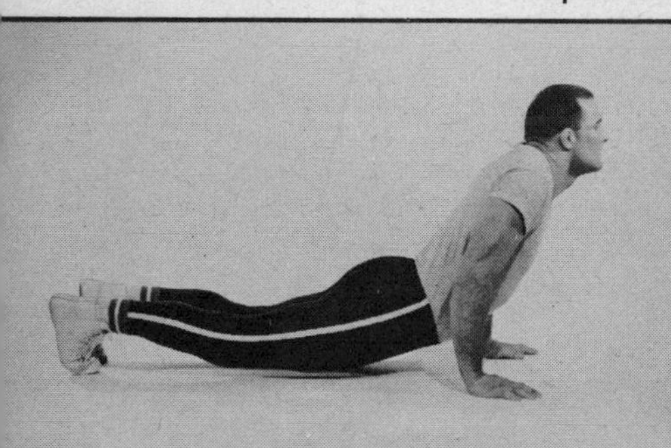

Start position: On floor, extend legs straight back and together, arms straight from shoulder to floor, back arched so hips almost touch floor.

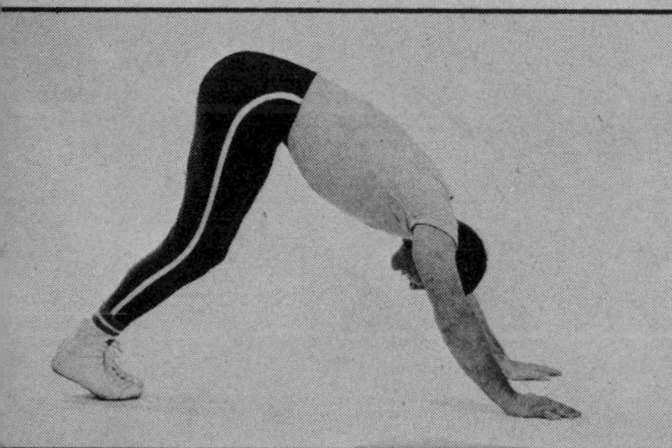

Action-Count 1. Raise hips as high as possible, at the same time push head down between arms.

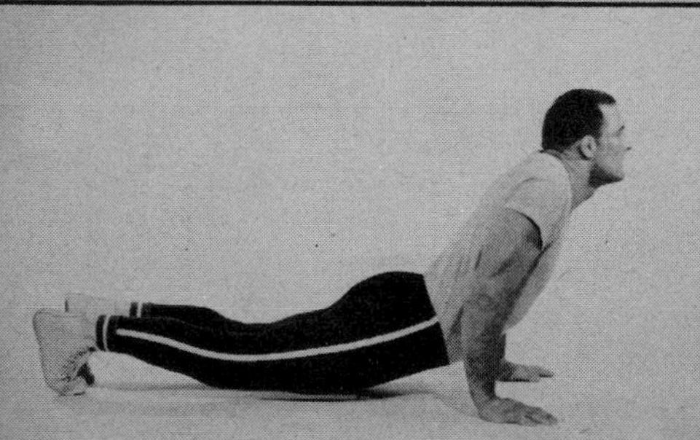

Count 2. Return to start position.

★ PRIMARY LEVEL

ISOMETRIC PERIOD

The isometric period of the total-fitness plan should start one minute after the end of the last exercise in the warm-up period.

In some of the exercises described in this section it is necessary to use a piece of cord or rope: clothesline, for instance, that is too strong for you to break. It should be about 8 to 9 feet in length. Tie the ends together, forming the rope into one loop. You might also keep a couple of handkerchiefs or a pair of work gloves handy in case pulling on the loop proves uncomfortable.

Place a watch or clock with a sweep-second hand within view so that you can time yourself during each exercise.

Before attempting isometric contractions, memorize and practice the following:

Breathing: Before each contraction, inhale to about three-quarters of your capacity. This breath must be held for the time it takes for a contraction. Each exercise in this period is 10 seconds long. At the end of a contraction, you exhale as you relax.

Exerting Maximum Effort: This may take a few moments to master and will vary with the strength of the individual. In applying force, pressure must be gradually increased after contact is made. There should be *no movement* except for the tensing of the muscles involved. After a contraction is begun, it should take 4 seconds to reach the point of maximum effort—the point beyond which pressure cannot be intensified and the muscles involved in the contraction start to quiver.

In each of the isometric contractions, the point of maximum effort should be held for 6 seconds. Coupled with the 4 seconds required to reach maximum effort, each exercise, then, lasts a total of 10 seconds.

Between each of the contractions there should be a 15-second rest period during which you prepare for the next exercise.

IT IS ONLY NECESSARY TO DO EACH EXERCISE ONCE to get maximum results.

Total time for this period: 6 minutes, 45 seconds.

Time all exercises with the seconds' hand of a clock.

★ **PRIMARY LEVEL**
Isometric #1
Time: 10 seconds

PARADE REST

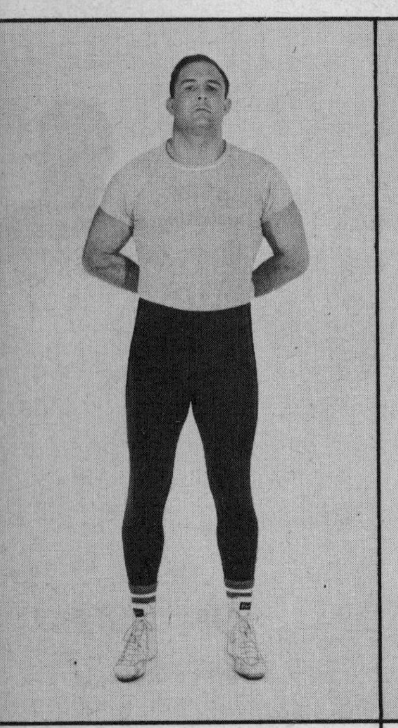

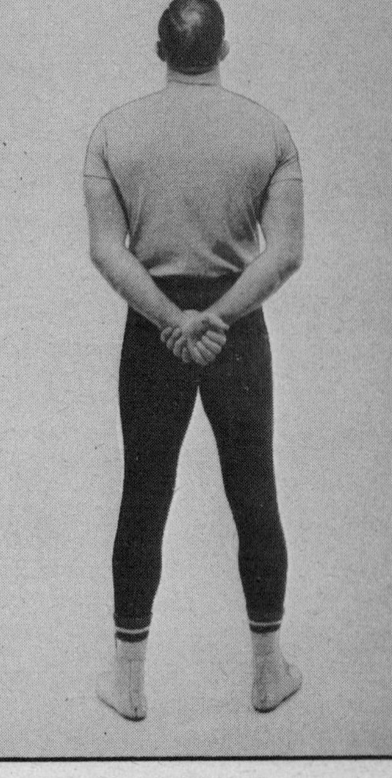

Start position: Stand erect, feet apart, chest raised, stomach flat. Place hands behind small of back and grasp right wrist with left hand. Inhale.

Contraction: Press backs of hands against small of back. Increase pressure of arms as if to pass hands through your body. Build up force for 4 seconds until maximum effort is reached. Hold maximum effort for 6 seconds. Relax and exhale.

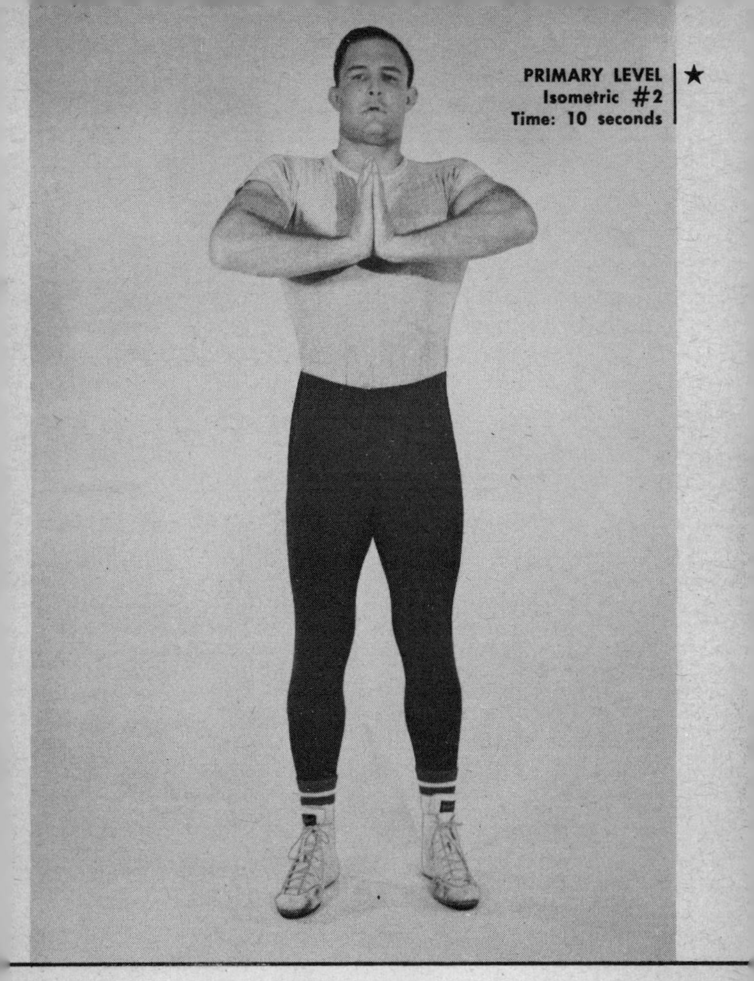

PALM PUSH

Start position: Stand erect, place palms of hands together in front of chest, fingers pointing up. Forearms form a straight line in front of chest.

Contraction: Inhale. Press palms together, keeping forearms in a straight line. Increase pressure for 4 seconds. Hold maximum effort for 6 seconds.
Relax and exhale.

★ **PRIMARY LEVEL**
Isometric #3
Time: 10 seconds

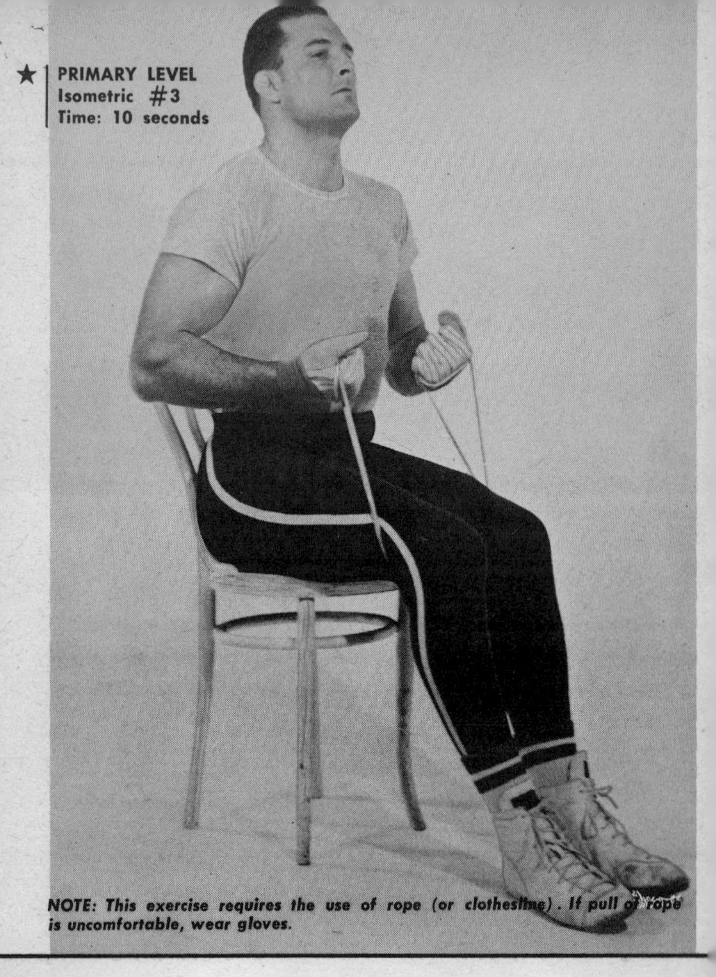

NOTE: This exercise requires the use of rope (or clothesline). If pull of rope is uncomfortable, wear gloves.

TWO-HAND CURL

Start position: Sit erect in a chair. Place rope under your legs behind knees, putting hands palms upward inside ends, as shown. Arms should be bent at elbow to form a right angle. (NOTE: If looped rope is too long, take a couple of turns around each hand until it is the desired length.)

Contraction: Inhale. Force palms up against loop, keeping feet flat on the floor. Increase pressure for 4 seconds. Hold maximum effort for 6 seconds.

Relax and exhale.

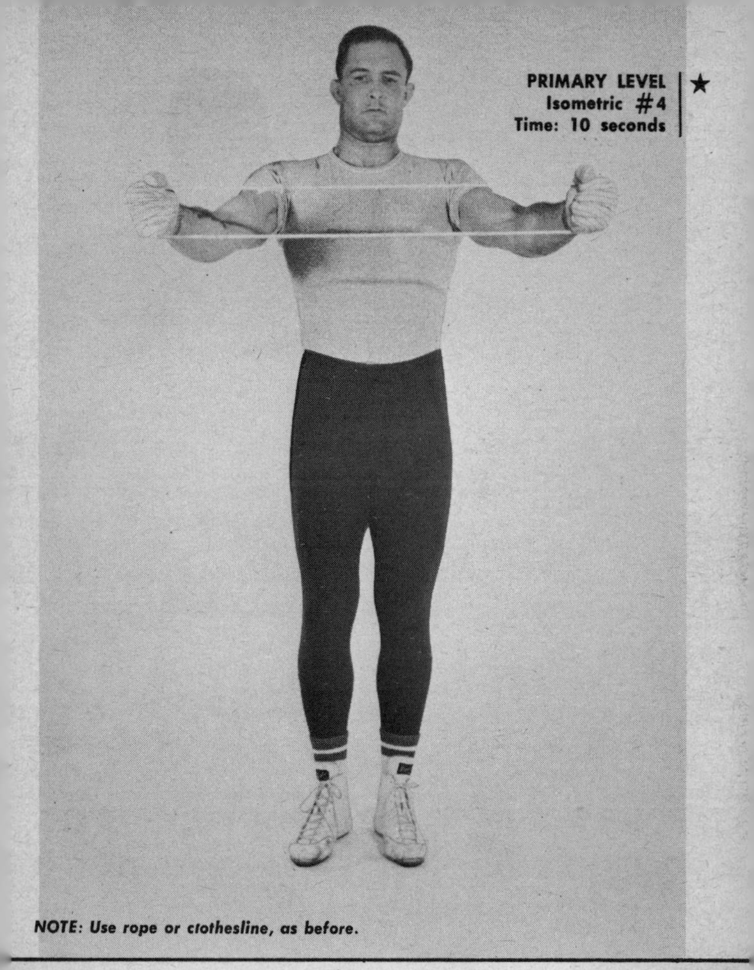

***NOTE**: Use rope or clothesline, as before.*

FRONT CABLE STRETCH

Start position: Stand erect, grasp looped rope at arms-length in front of chest, palms facing.

Contraction: Inhale. Pull apart on loop, increasing effort for 4 seconds. Keep elbows straight. Hold maximum effort for 6 seconds.

Relax and exhale.

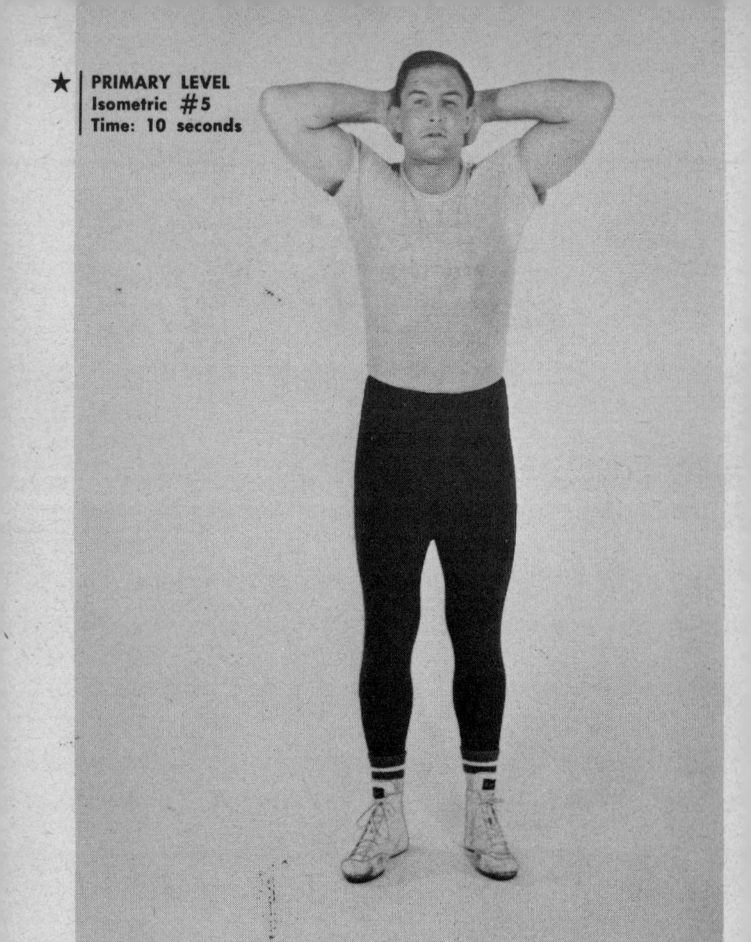

NECK PRESS

Start position: Stand erect. Place hands behind head, fingers interlaced, upper arms parallel, elbows forward.

Contraction: Inhale. Force hands forward against back of head.

Keep head rigid by pushing back against hands. Increase pressure for 4 seconds. Hold maximum effort for 6 seconds.

Relax and exhale.

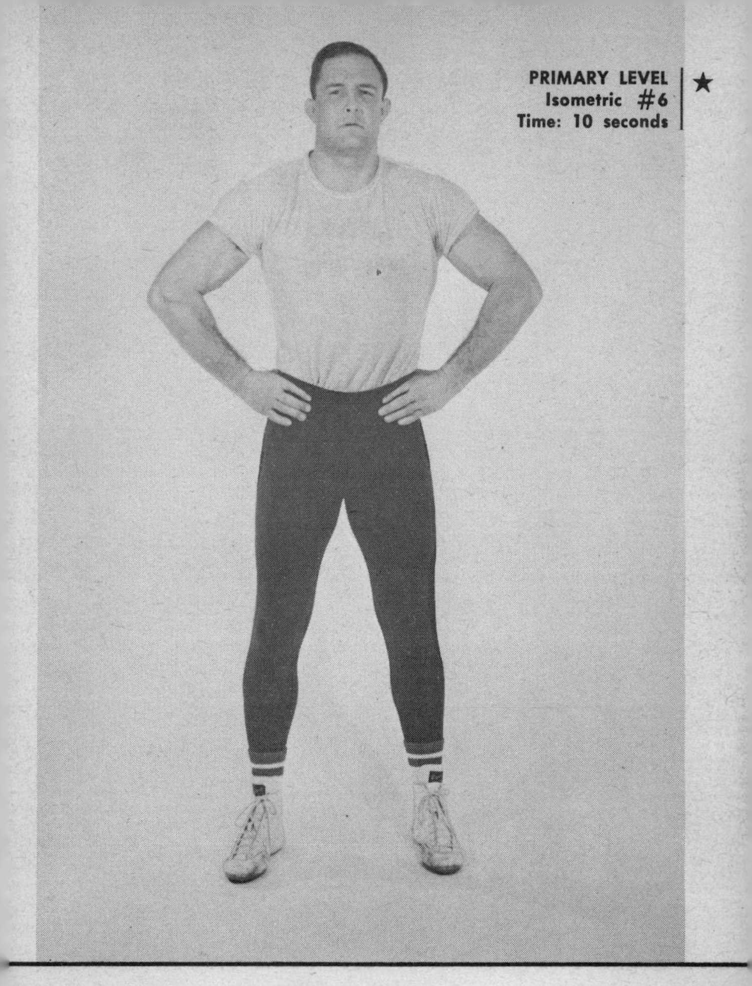

HIP PRESS

Start position: Stand erect, hands on hip bones, fingers to front.

Contraction: Inhale. Press hands against hips as if to bring them together through torso. Increase pressure for 4 seconds. Hold maximum effort for 6 seconds.

Relax and exhale.

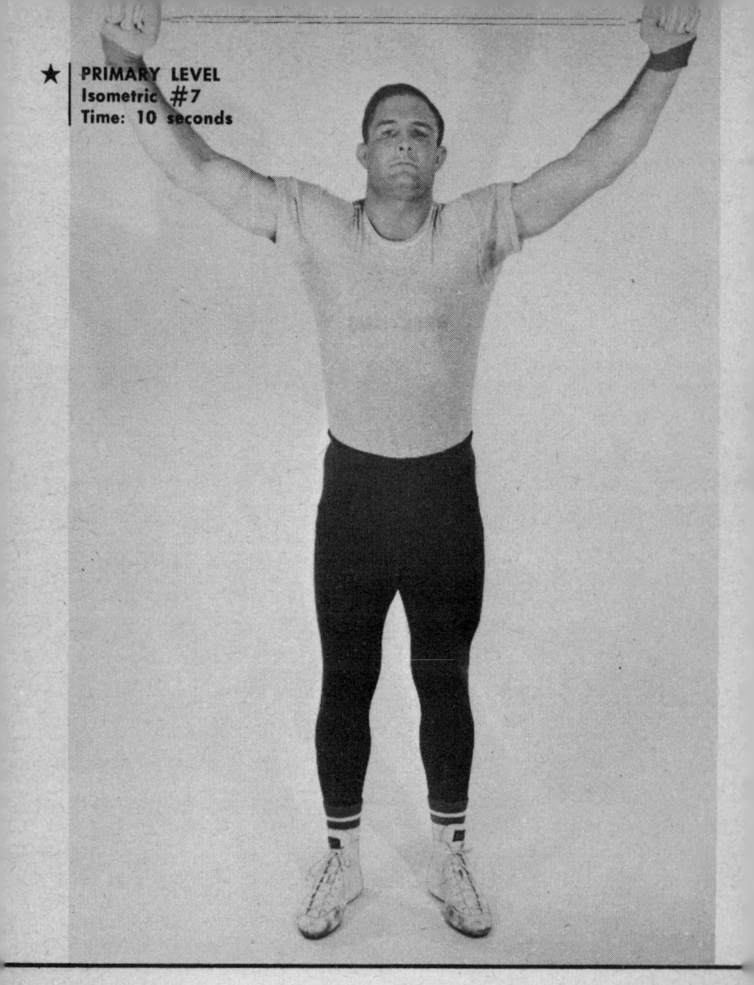

OVERHEAD CABLE STRETCH

Start position: Stand erect. Hold loop overhead, arms straight, palms outward. (Take up length of loop by turning around each hand one time.)

Contraction: Inhale. Force arms outward, attempting to pull loop apart. Increase pressure for 4 seconds. Hold maximum effort 6 seconds.

Relax and exhale.

NOTE: *This exercise requires the use of rope (or clothesline) as previously described. If pull of rope is uncomfortable, wear gloves.*

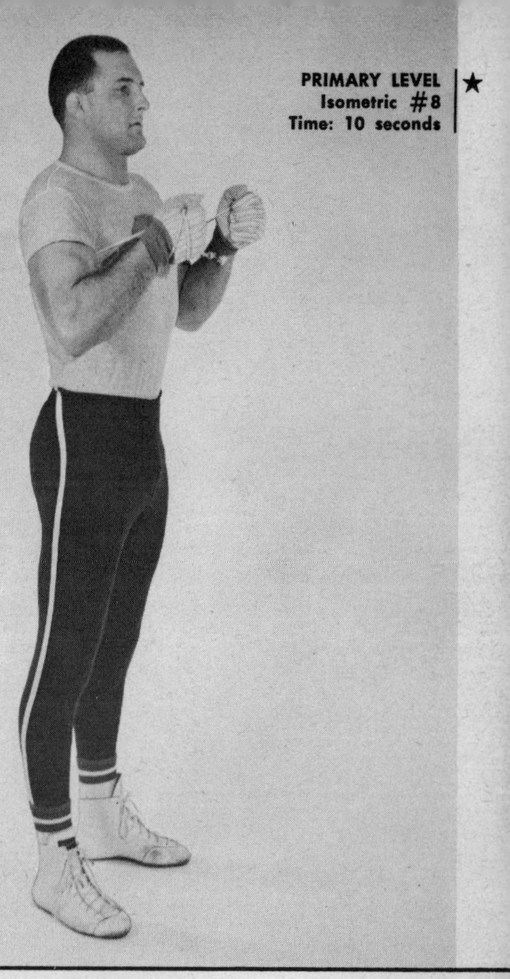

TRICEPS PUSH

Start position: Stand erect, place loop around back under arms, at elbow height. Bend arms and grasp ends of loop palms facing away.

Contraction: Inhale. Push arms forward while pressing against rope with back. Increase pressure for 4 seconds. Hold maximum effort for 6 seconds.

Relax and exhale.

***NOTE:** This exercise requires the use of rope (or clothesline) as previously described. If pull of rope is uncomfortable, wear gloves.*

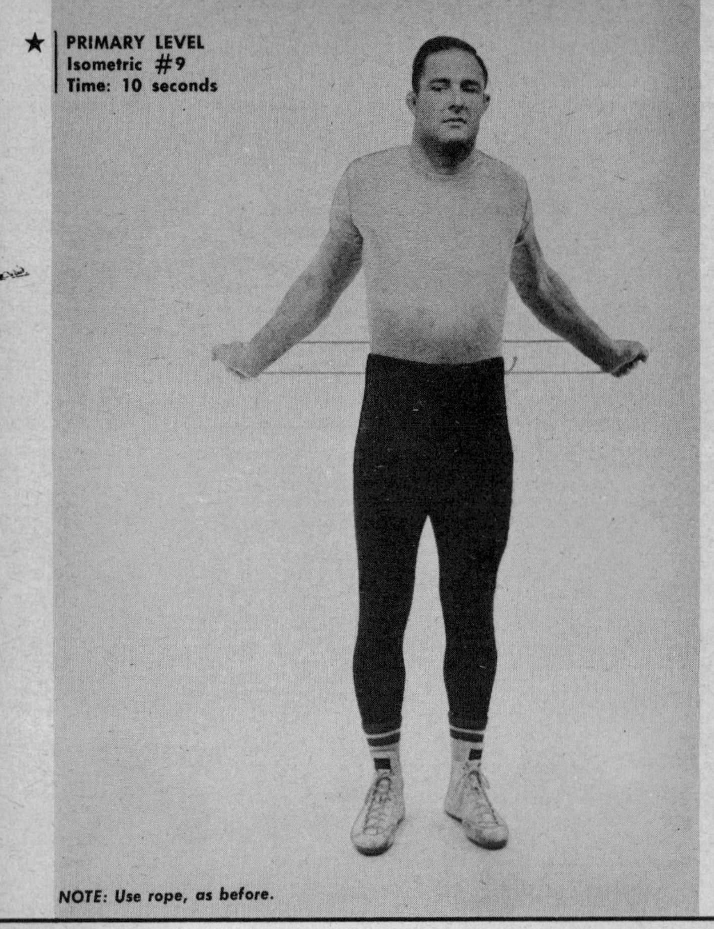

NOTE: Use rope, as before.

BACK CABLE STRETCH

Position: Adjust loop to about 3 feet in length. Stand erect with loop behind the small of your back. Grasp ends of loop with both hands, palms facing outward.

Contraction: Inhale. Pull outward, attempting to pull loop apart. Increase effort for 4 seconds. Hold maximum effort for 6 seconds.

Relax and exhale.

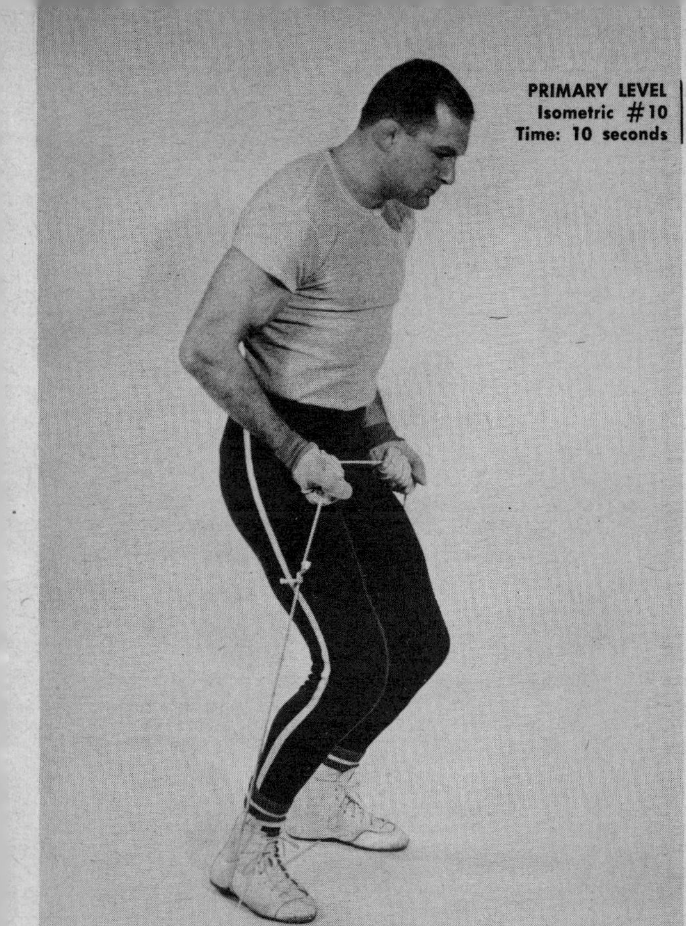

***NOTE:** Use rope (or clothesline) as before.*

DEAD LIFT

Start position: Stand with both feet on inside of loop. Grasp loop at sides with both hands, palms up. Assume semi-squat position with back straight. Take up slack in loop by winding excess rope around hands.

Contraction: Inhale. Using legs and back, attempt to come erect against resistance of loop. Increase pressure for 4 seconds. Hold maximum effort for 6 seconds.

Relax and exhale.

★ PRIMARY LEVEL

ISOTONIC PERIOD

The *isotonic* period begins as soon as you have completed the isometric period. These exercises are included to condition the muscles and also to strengthen the heart and improve circulation.

As total fitness improves and you are able to do more, the number of repetitions will gradually increase.

Practice the exercises a few times to get the rhythm of executing them properly through every count. When exercising against time there is a tendency to go through the movements sloppily, sliding from one count to the next. The timing for these exercises was prepared so that the count is done smartly. Once the coordinations are mastered the exercises can be done with ease.

There should be no rest between exercises at this level except the time it takes to go from one position to the next.

Total time for this period: approximately 3 minutes.

PRIMARY LEVEL ★
Isotonic #1
Time: 15-30 seconds*

JUMPING JACK

12 times, First and Second Weeks
24 times, Third Week

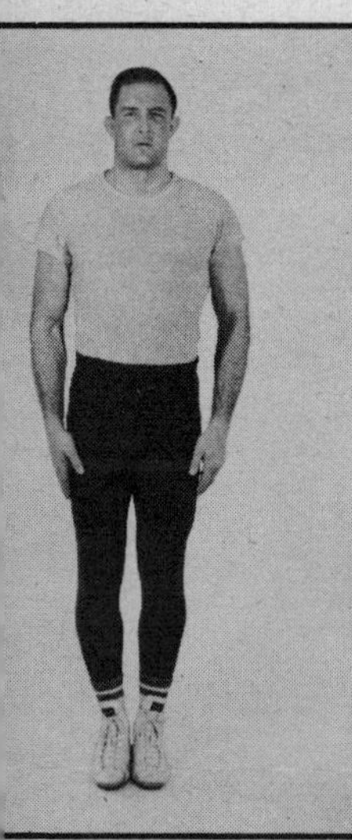

Start position: Stand erect, hands at sides, legs together.

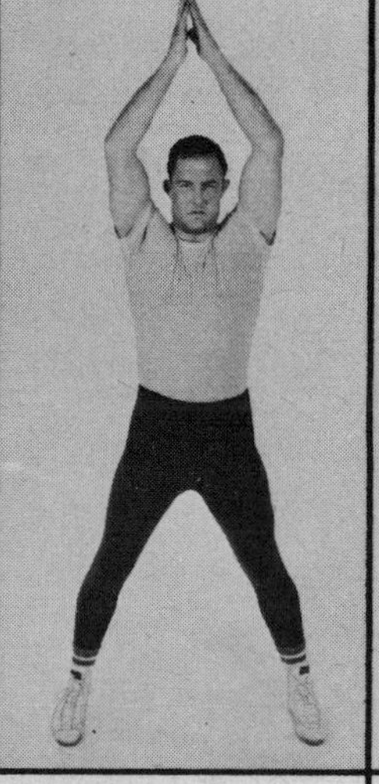

Action-Count 1. Jump to legs apart, simultaneously raising arms overhead, sidewards, elbows straight, and clap hands together.

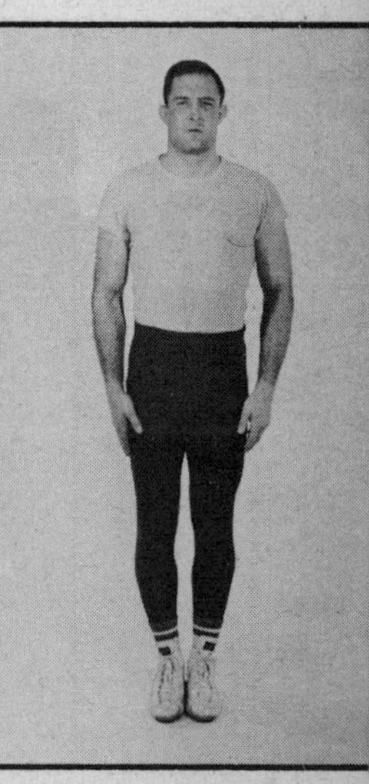

Count 2. Return by jumping to start position.

****15 seconds, First and Second Weeks***
****30 seconds, Third Week***

★ **PRIMARY LEVEL**
Isotonic #2
Time: 30 seconds

FRONT WAIST BEND

12 times, First and Second Weeks
15 times, Third Week

Start position: Sit on floor, arms clasped behind neck, fingers interlaced, legs extended to front and apart.

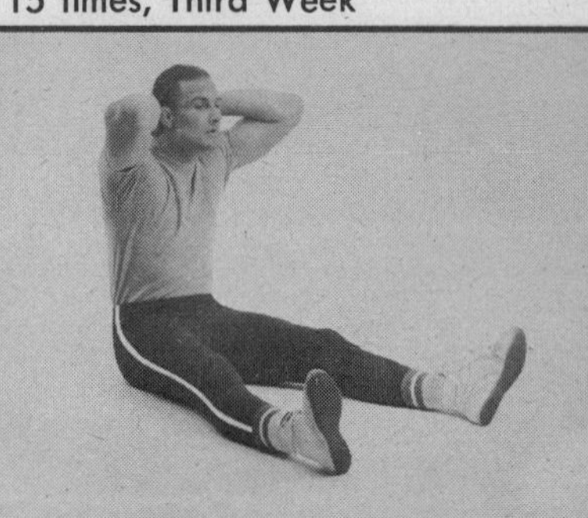

Action-Count 1. Bend trunk forward until elbows touch knees. Keep knees as straight as possible.

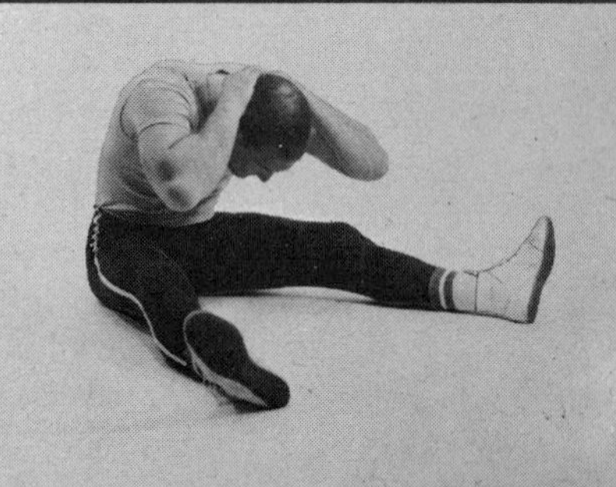

Count 2. Return to start position.

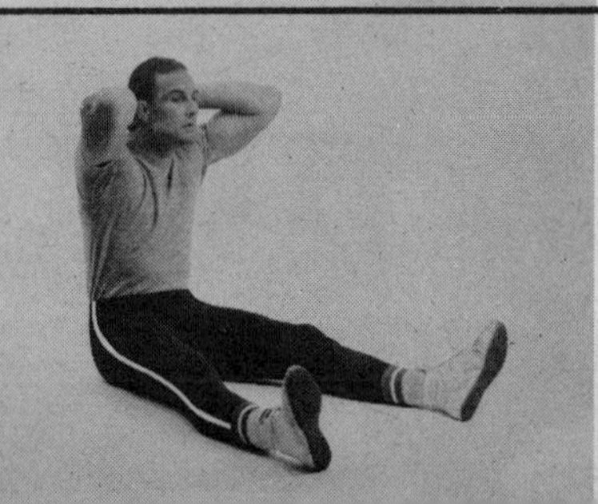

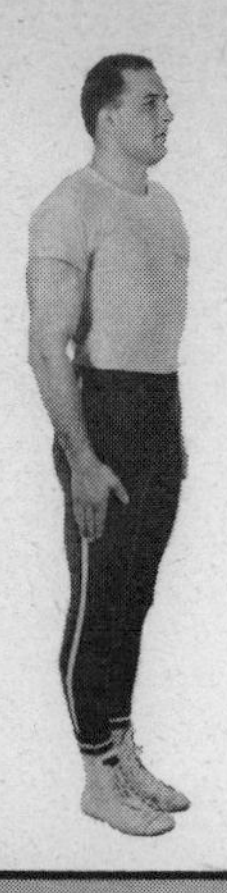

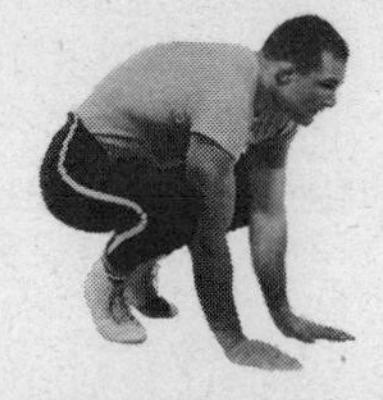

PRIMARY LEVEL ★
Isotonic #3
Time: 30 seconds

SQUAT THRUST

10 times, First and Second Weeks
12 times, Third Week

Start Position: Stand erect, legs together, arms at sides.

Action-Count 1. Squat, placing hands flat on floor, elbows straight.

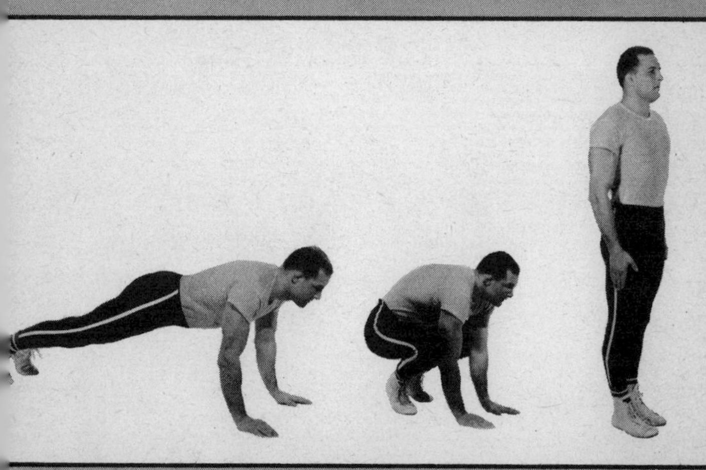

Count 2. Throw both legs straight backwards to extended position.

Count 3. Jump back to squat position as in Count 2.

Count 4. Return to start position.

★ **PRIMARY LEVEL**
Isotonic #4
Time: 25-30 seconds*

KNEE PUSH-UPS

10 times, First and Second Weeks
14 times, Third Week

Start Position: Lie prone on floor, elbows bent, hands flat on floor at chest.

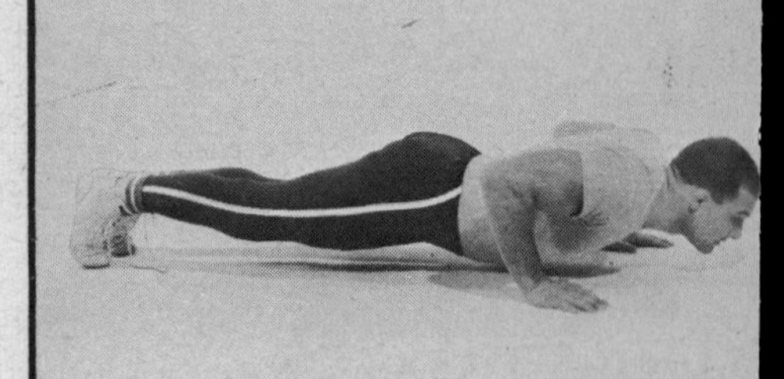

Action-Count 1. Push chest straight off floor to arms-length. Bend knees as you go up and rest on them.

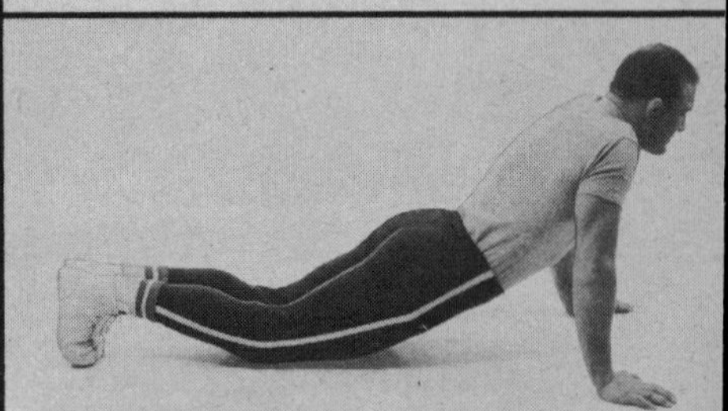

Count 2. Return to start position.

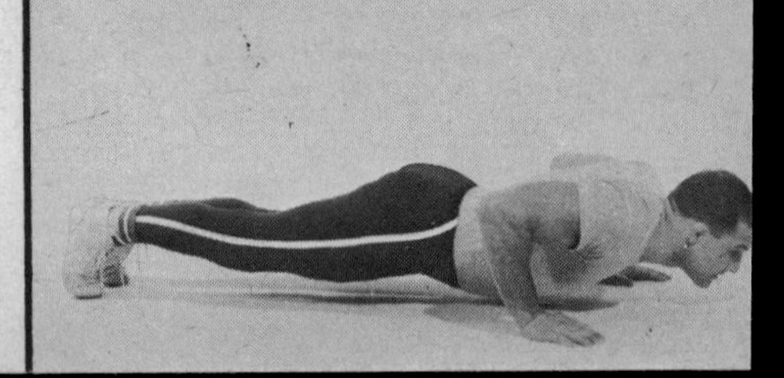

****25 seconds, First and Second Weeks***
****30 seconds, Third Week***

PRIMARY LEVEL ★
Isotonic #5
Time: 30-45 seconds*

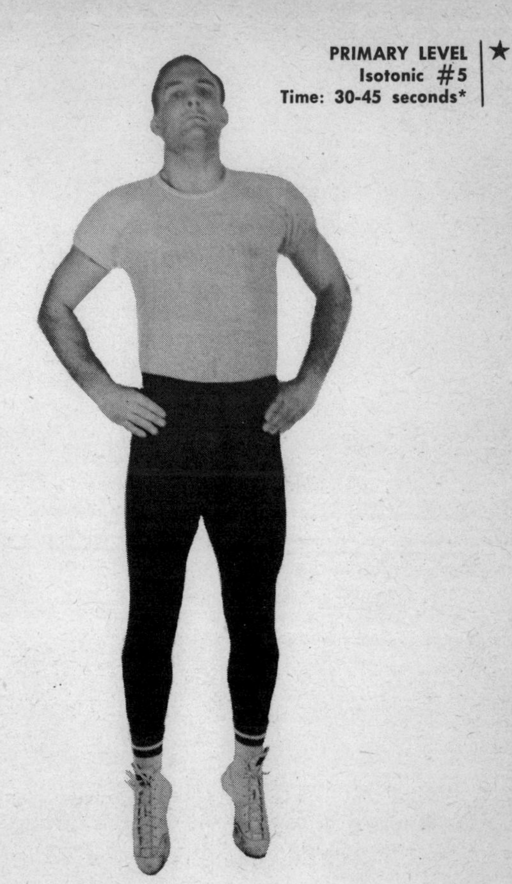

**30 seconds, First and Second Weeks*
**45 seconds, Third Week*

IMAGINARY ROPE SKIP

60 times, First and Second Weeks
90 times, Third Week

Hop in place for allotted time, clearing floor with enough height to go over an imaginary rope. (Some exercisers find this easier to do if they turn their wrists while hopping as if rope skipping.) Keep count throughout and time this exercise accurately.

★ ★ SECONDARY LEVEL

The Secondary Level is designed for those who have completed the Primary Level and desire a more vigorous program.

Progressing through the following two charts of the Secondary Level will help insure your total fitness. The results will enable you to live a more vigorous life, to participate more fully in sports, and provide the stamina needed in times of unusual exertion.

It is not necessary for one to proceed beyond the Secondary Level to maintain a good degree of total fitness. If, however, you wish to attain an unusually high level of fitness, or to call upon that fitness in competitive athletics, you should go on to the Peak Level after completing the Secondary.

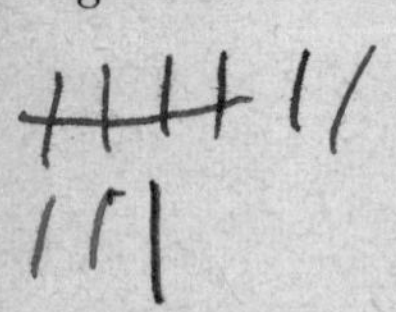

★ ★ SECONDARY LEVEL

CHART I

Fourth & Fifth Weeks
Follow this chart for two weeks
before proceeding to Secondary Level Chart II

	Exercise	Repetitions	Time in Secs
WARM-UP	1. Stretch and Bend	12	30
	2. Squat and Touch	10	30
	3. Knee-Hug	10	30
	4. Twist and Touch	10	45
	5. Seal Bend	10	40
ISOMETRIC	1. Doorway Press	1	10
	2. Lateral Raise	1	10
	3. Knee Pull	1	10
	4. Knee Press (Interior)	1	10
	5. Knee Press (Exterior)	1	10
	6. Abdominal Contraction	1	10
	7. Dead Lift	1	10
	8. Under Leg Curl	1	10
	9. Toe Raise	1	10
	10. Toe Pull	1	10
ISOTONIC	1. Jumping Jack	30	30
	2. Sit-Up	8	30
	3. Squat Thrust	14	30
	4. Push-Up	15	30
	5. Rope Skipping	120	1-min.

CHART II

Sixth and Seventh Weeks

	Exercise	Repetitions	Time in Secs
WARM-UP	1. Stretch and Bend	12	30
	2. Squat and Touch	10	30
	3. Knee-Hug	10	30
	4. Twist and Touch	10	45
	5. Seal Bend	10	40
ISOMETRIC	1. Doorway Press	1	10
	2. Lateral Raise	1	10
	3. Knee Pull	1	10
	4. Knee Press (Interior)	1	10
	5. Knee Press (Exterior)	1	10
	6. Abdominal Contraction	1	10
	7. Dead Lift	1	10
	8. Under Leg Curl	1	10
	9. Toe Raise	1	10
	10. Toe Pull	1	10
ISOTONIC	1. Jumping Jack	45	45
	2. Sit-Up	10	30
	3. Squat Thrust	15	30
	4. Push-Up	20	30
	5. Rope Skipping	175	1-min. 30 secs.

★ ★ SECONDARY LEVEL

WARM-UP PERIOD

The following *five* exercises must *always* be done before going into the isometric-isotonic period.

They are identical to those in the Primary Level. You need not increase the number of repetitions nor shorten the time of execution. These will prepare you adequately for the two periods that follow.

BEND AND STRETCH

This exercise should be repeated *12 times.*

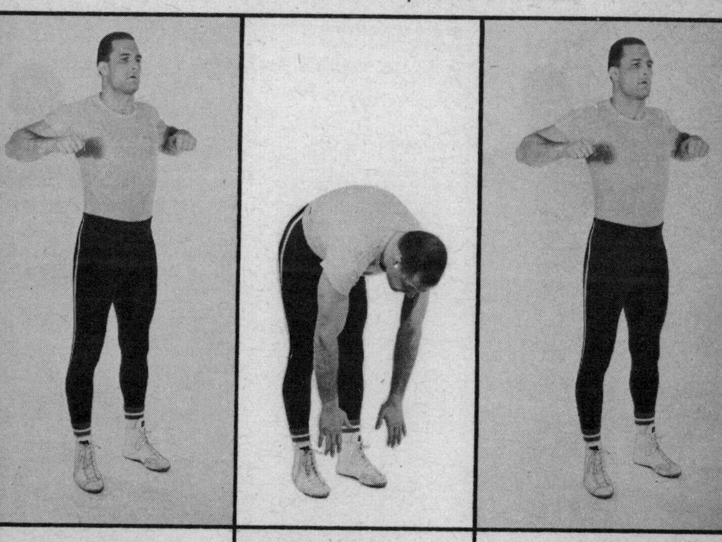

Start position: Stand erect, arms at shoulder level, fists clenched, elbows bent and thrust back as far as possible.

Action-Count 1. Bend forward to floor, with arms hanging down and fingers relaxed. Bend knees slightly and allow head to hang forward.

Count 2. Return to start position.

★★ **SECONDARY LEVEL**
Warm-up #2
Time: 30 seconds

SQUAT AND TOUCH

This exercise should be repeated *10 times.*

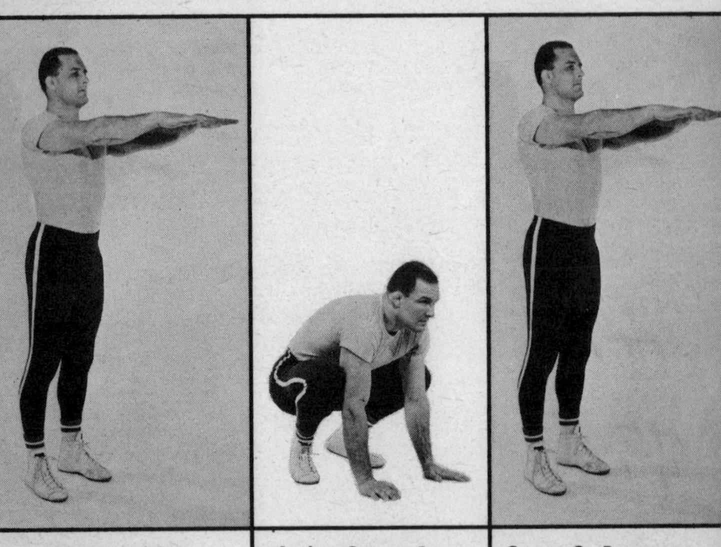

Start position: Stand erect, arms extended to front, palms down, feet about 12 inches apart.

Action-Count 1. Bend knees and squat, touching fingers or palms of hands to floor between knees. Keep head erect and back straight.

Count 2. Return to start position.

SECONDARY LEVEL ★
Warm-up #3 ★
Time: 30 seconds

KNEE-HUG

This exercise should be repeated *10 times*, and each repetition represents 4 counts.

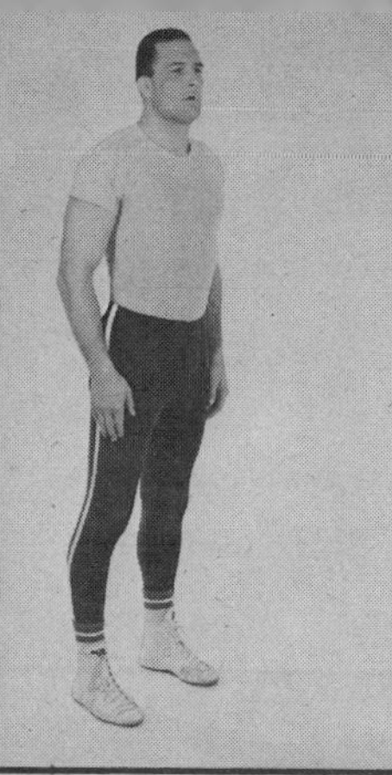

Start position: Stand erect, back straight, arms at sides.

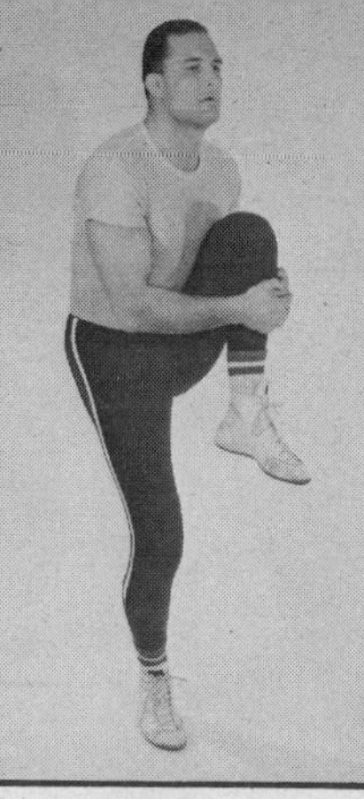

Action-Count 1. Raise left knee to chest level. Grasp lower leg with both arms and draw leg to chest. Keep back straight.

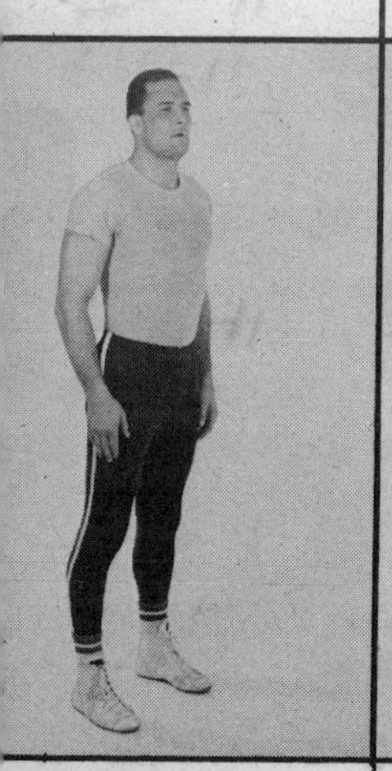

Count 2. Return to start position.

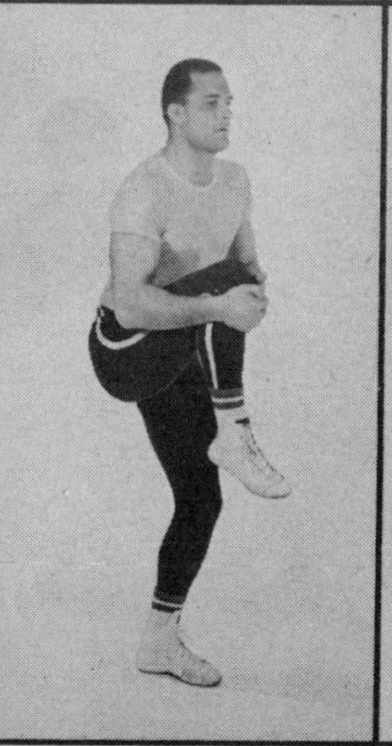

Count 3. Raise right knee to chest as in Count 1.

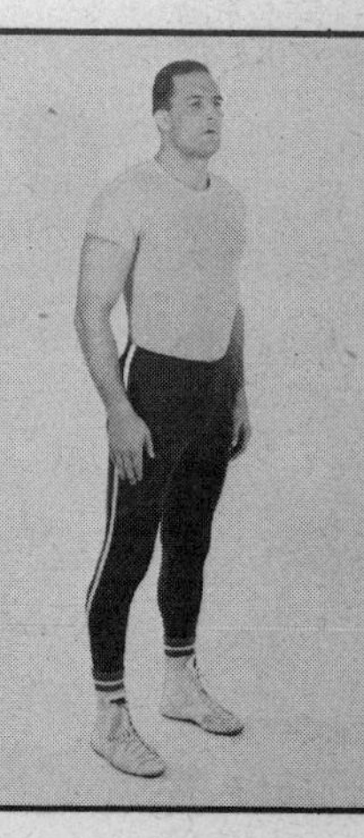

Count 4. Return to start position.

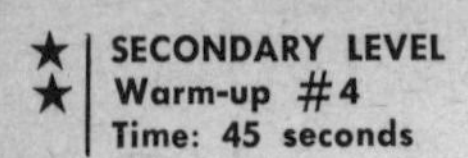

TWIST AND TOUCH

This exercise should be repeated *10 times,* and each repetition represents 4 counts.

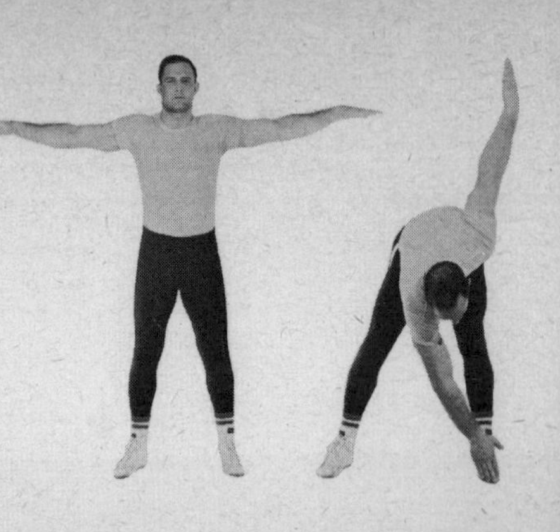

Start position: Stand erect, arms extended at sides, palms down, legs apart

Action-Count 1. Twist to left, touching right fingertips to left toe, extending left arm vertically. (Left knee may be slightly bent.)

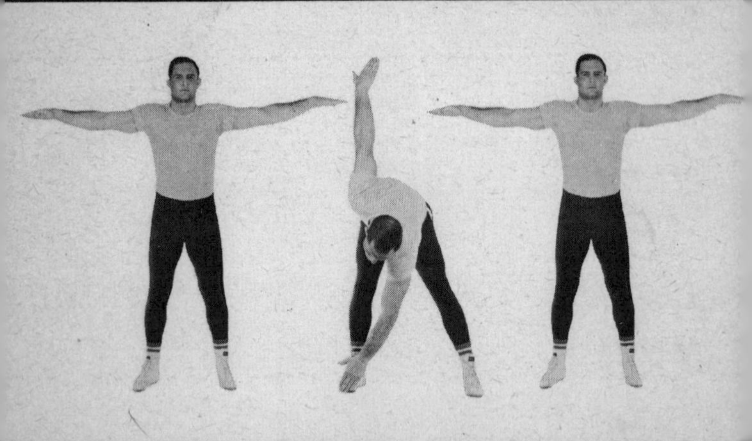

Count 2. Return to start position.

Count 3. Raise right knee to chest as in Count 1.

Count 4. Return to start position.

SEAL BEND

This exercise should be repeated *10 times.*

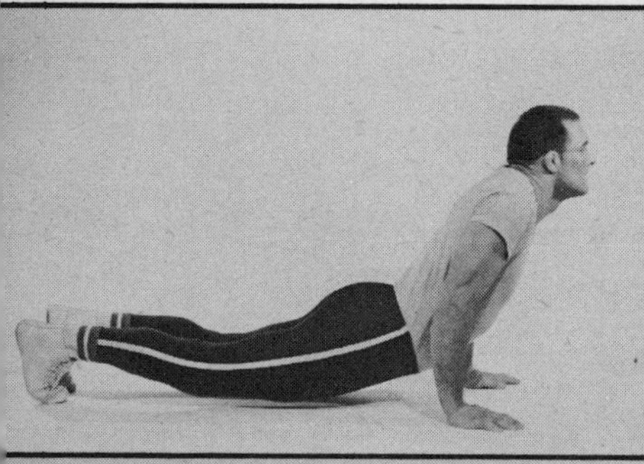

Start position: On floor, extend legs straight back and together, arms straight from shoulder to floor, back arched so hips almost touch floor.

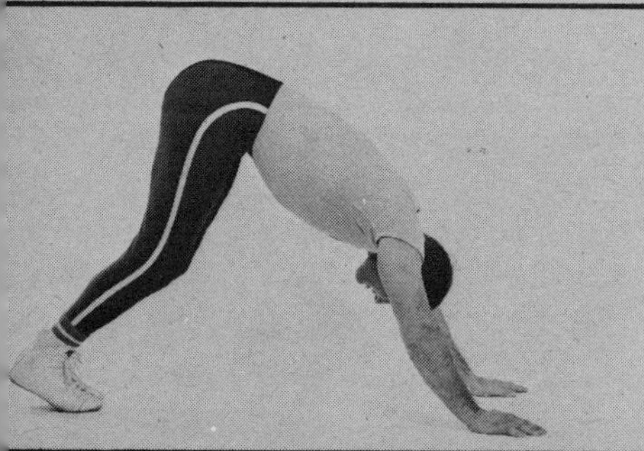

Action-Count 1. Raise hips as high as possible, at the same time push head down between arms.

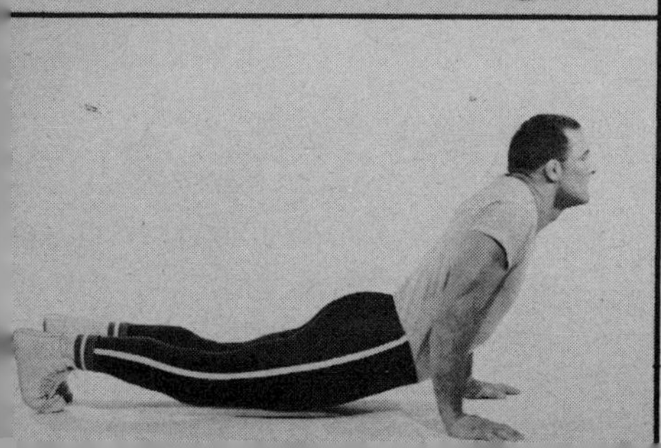

Count 2. Return to start position.

★ ★ SECONDARY LEVEL

ISOMETRIC PERIOD

This period begins *one minute after* the warm-up period.

The contractions allow larger muscle groups in the body to act in concert to provide massive concentration of effort. They should not be attempted with maximum effort until you have mastered *all* the exercises at the Primary Level.

The time allotted for each exercise remains at 10 seconds (the ideal time element for isometric contractions) and each exercise should be done *once only*.

Additional equipment needed for this series of exercises: a strong broomstick about 30 inches long.

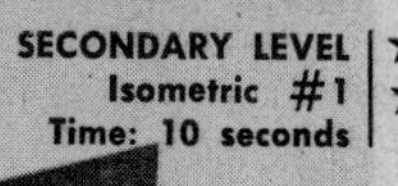

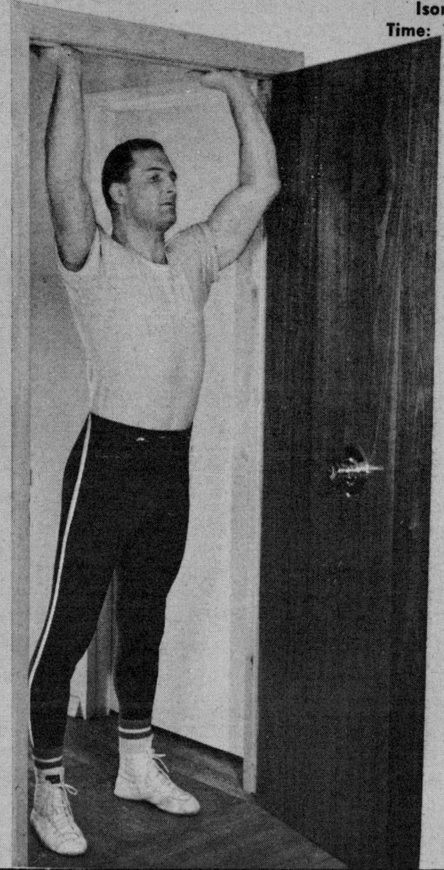

DOORWAY PRESS

Position: Stand erect in doorway. Place palms of hands on top of doorway, arms bent halfway. (If you do not reach the top of door stand on some books or ther solid base until you do.)

Contraction: Inhale. Using arms and back, press upward with palms of hands against top of door. Increase pressure for 4 seconds until maximum effort is reached. Hold maximum effort for 6 seconds.

Relax and exhale.

★★ SECONDARY LEVEL
Isometric #2
Time: 10 seconds

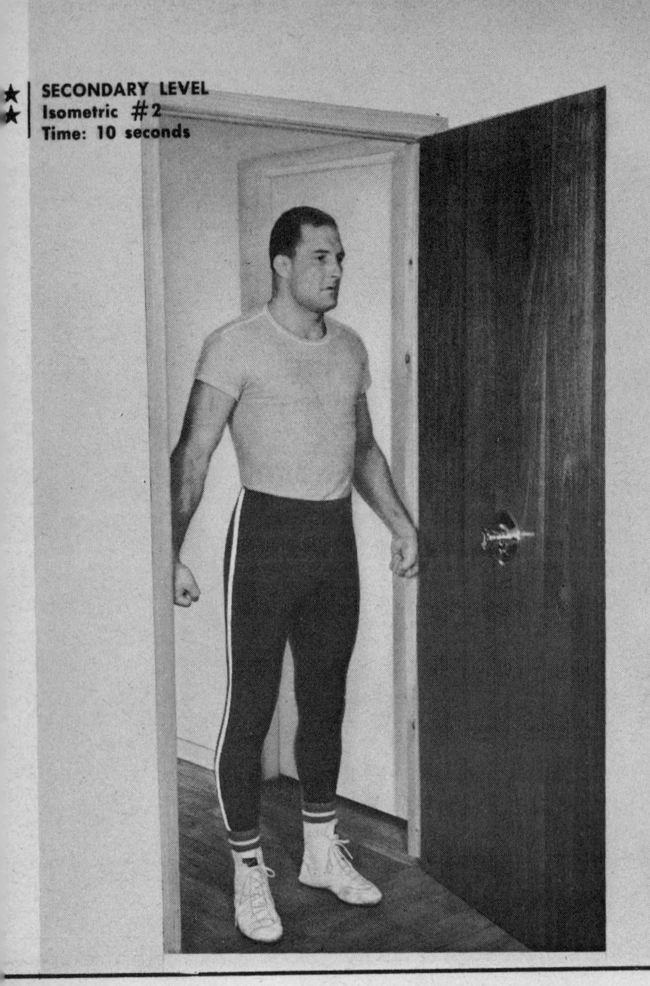

LATERAL RAISE

Position: Stand erect in doorway. Place backs of hands against sides of door, touching on both sides.

Contraction: Inhale. Attempt to raise both arms simultaneously upward and sideward. Increase pressure for 4 seconds until maximum effort is reached. Hold maximum effort for 6 seconds.

Relax and exhale.

SECONDARY LEVEL ★
Isometric #3 ★
Time: 10 seconds

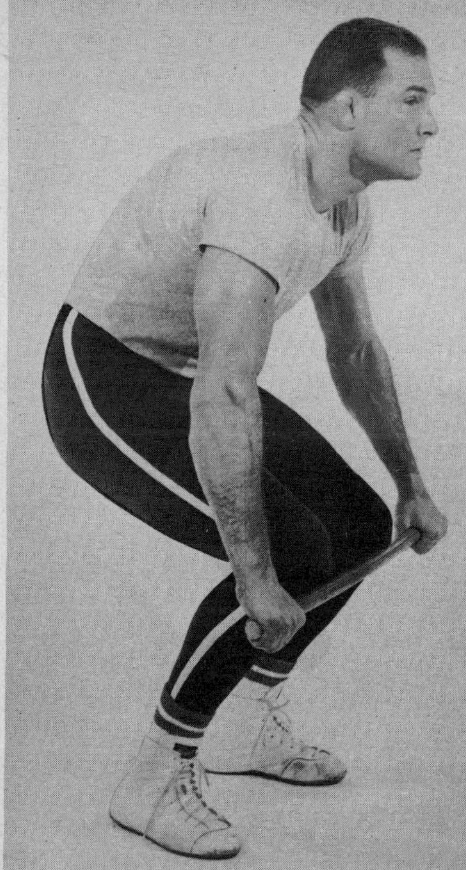

NOTE: This exercise requires the use of a 30-inch broomstick.

KNEE PULL

Position: Semi-squat. Place broomstick in front of knees. (Place knees as close to ends of stick as possible, allowing enough of stick to extend at either end for firm grasp.)

Contraction: Inhale. Pull backward and upward, with back and arms against broomstick. Increase pressure for 4 seconds. Hold maximum effort for 6 seconds.

Relax and exhale.

★★ **SECONDARY LEVEL**
Isometric #4
Time: 10 seconds

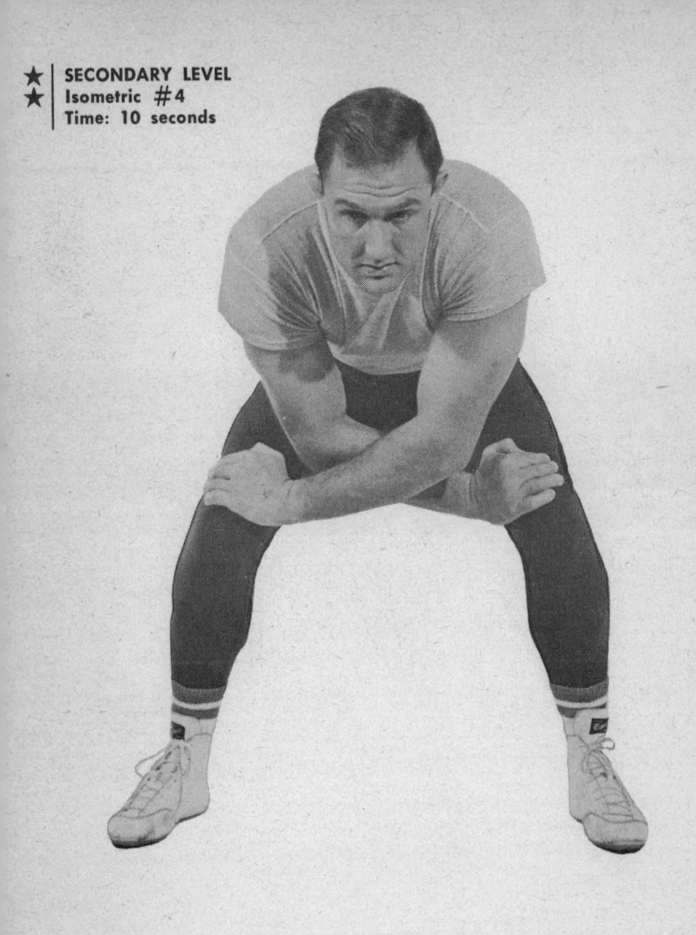

KNEE-PRESS (INTERIOR)

Position: Semi-squat forward, cross arms and place palms of hands against *insides* of opposite knees.

Contraction: Inhale. Press palms outward against insides of knees and simultaneously try to force knees together. Increase effort for 4 seconds until maximum effort is reached. Hold maximum effort for 6 seconds.

Relax and exhale.

SECONDARY LEVEL ★★
Isometric #5
Time: 10 seconds

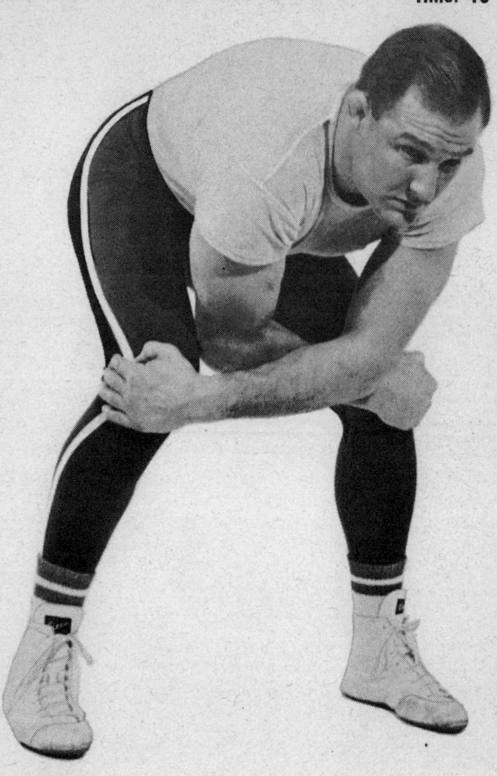

KNEE PRESS (EXTERIOR)

Position: Semi-squat forward. Cross arms and grasp outside of opposite knees.

Contraction: Inhale. Attempt to pull knees together with hands, at the same time force knees apart with legs. Increase effort for 4 seconds and hold maximum effort for 6 seconds.

Relax and exhale.

SECONDARY LEVEL
Isometric #6
Time: 10 seconds

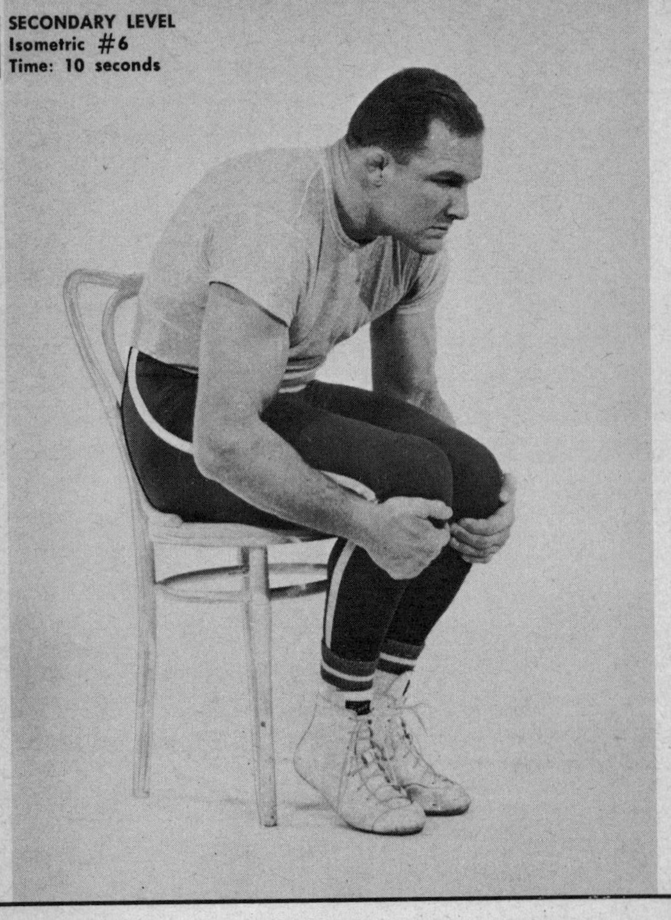

ABDOMINAL CONTRACTION AND HEEL PRESS

Position: Sit in chair, legs together, heels raised off floor. Lean forward and grasp both knees with hands.

Contraction: Inhale. Tense stomach, attempt to force heels to floor. At the same time, pull back on knees so that heels cannot be lowered. Increase force of action for 4 seconds. Hold maximum effort for 6 seconds.

Relax and exhale.

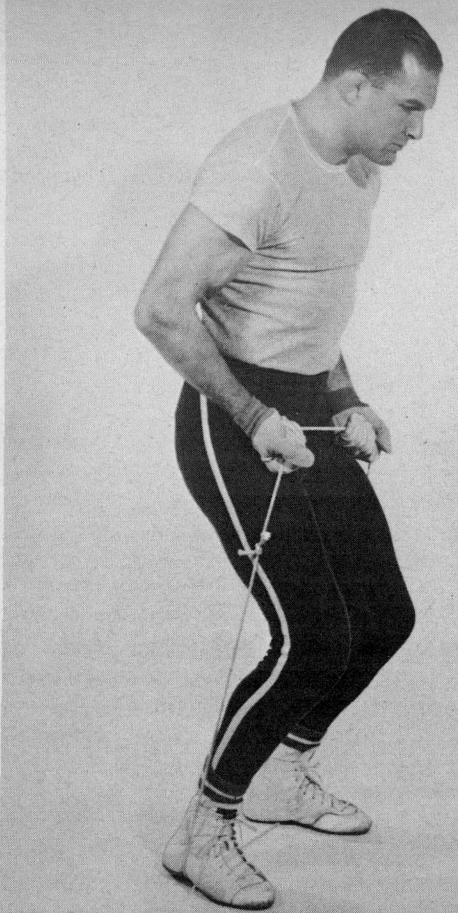

SECONDARY LEVEL ★★
Isometric #7
Time: 10 seconds

***NOTE:** This exercise requires the use of a rope (or clothesline) as before.*

DEAD LIFT

Position: Stand with both feet within loop. Grasp loop at sides with both hands, palms up. Assume semi-squat position with back straight. Take up slack in loop by winding excess rope around hands.

Contraction: Inhale. Using legs and back, attempt to come erect against resistance of loop. Increase pressure for 4 seconds. Hold maximum effort for 6 seconds.
Relax and exhale.

★★ SECONDARY LEVEL
Isometric #8
Time: 10 seconds

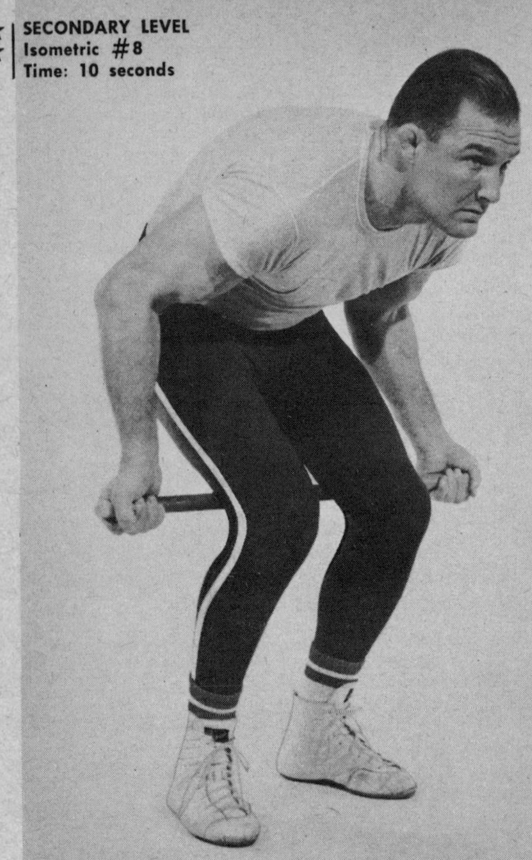

Note: This exercise requires the use of a 30-inch broomstick.

UNDER LEG CURL

Position: Place stick behind knees, grasping both ends with palms up. Assume semi-squat position.

Contraction: Inhale. Curl arms forward and upward, increasing pressure for 4 seconds. Hold maximum effort for 6 seconds.

Relax and exhale.

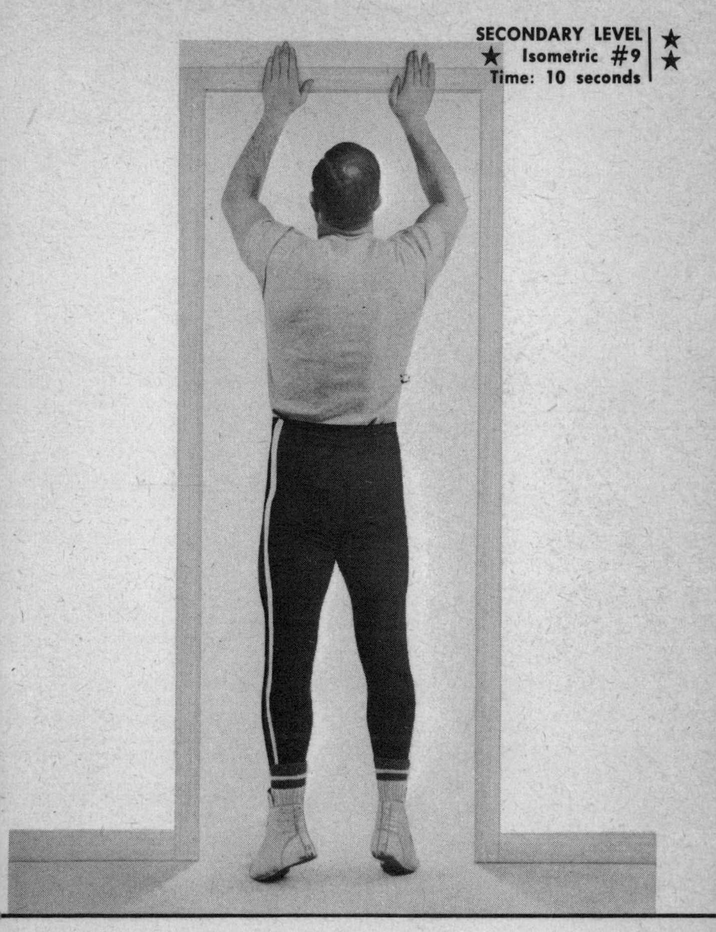

DOORWAY TOE RAISE

Position: Stand in doorway with palms of hands against top of doorway, arms extended. Raise up on toes until heels are off floor about one inch.

Contraction: Inhale. Push against top of doorway with arms straight so heels go back to floor, at the same time push back with calves of legs so that heels stay up. Increase pressure for 4 seconds. Hold maximum effort for 6 seconds.

Relax and exhale.

★★ **SECONDARY LEVEL**
Isometric #10
Time: 10 seconds

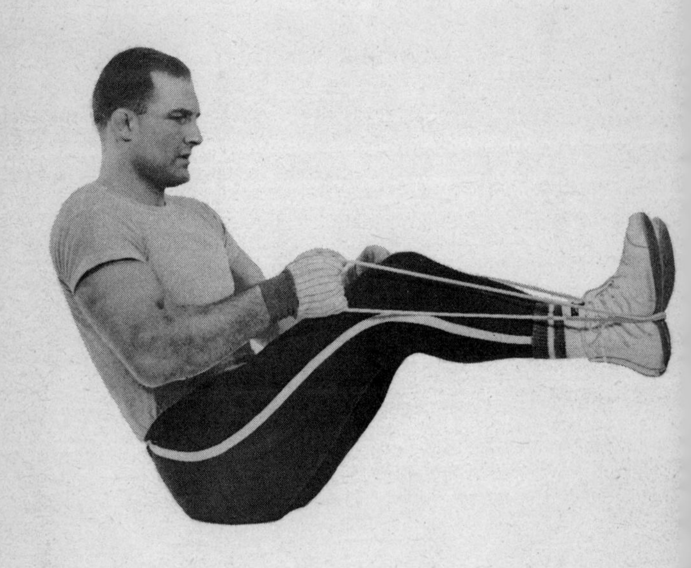

NOTE: This exercise requires the use of rope (or clothesline) as before.

TOE PULL

Position: Sit on floor, both sides of loop under feet, grasping end of loop with both hands. Lift legs off floor so lower leg is parallel with floor.

Contraction: Inhale. Attempt to extend both legs while restraining with arms. Increase pressure for 4 seconds until maximum effort attained. Hold maximum effort for 6 seconds.

Relax and exhale.

★ ★ SECONDARY LEVEL

ISOTONIC PERIOD

The following period requires more speed and more repetitions.

The total time allotted is extended by only one minute over the Primary Level, but the number of repetitions are increased.

Exercises #2 and #4 change in this period. The others remain the same.

Time each exercise carefully and execute each movement correctly.

★★ **SECONDARY LEVEL**
Isotonic #1
Time: 30-45 seconds*

JUMPING JACK

This exercise should be repeated:
30 times, Fourth and Fifth Weeks
45 times, Sixth and Seventh Weeks

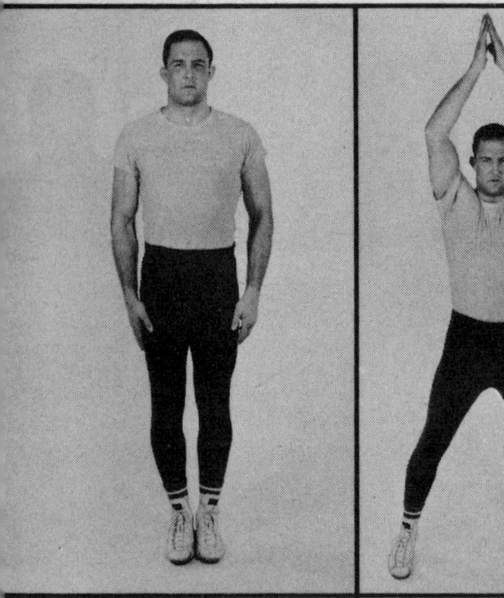

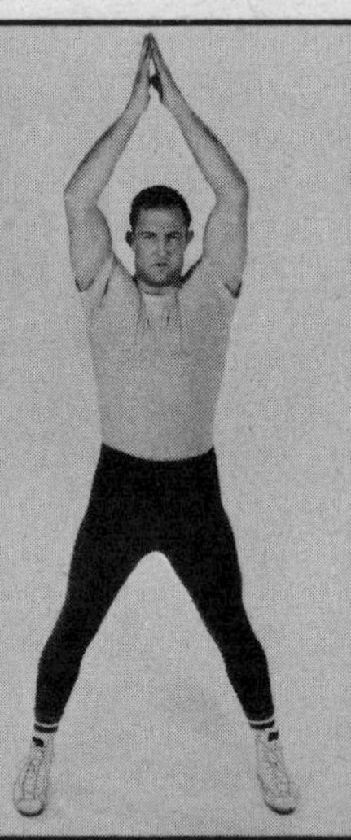

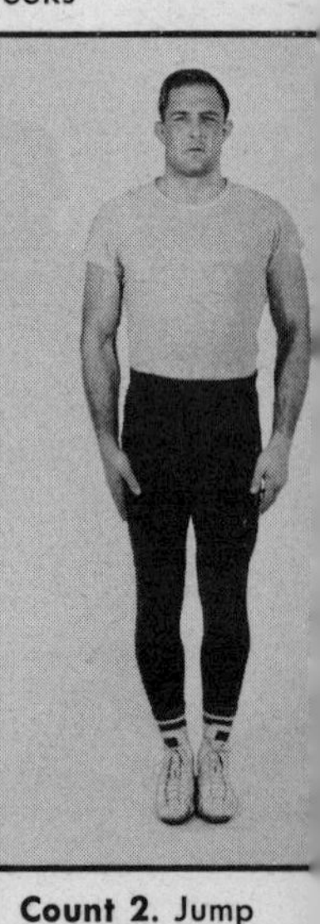

Start Position: Stand erect hands at side, legs together.

Action-Count 1. Jump to legs apart, simultaneously raising arms sidewards overhead, elbows straight, and clap hands.

Count 2. Jump back to start position.

****30 seconds, Fourth and Fifth Weeks***
****45 seconds, Sixth and Seventh Weeks***

SIT-UPS

This exercise should be repeated:
8 times, Fourth and Fifth Weeks
10 times, Sixth and Seventh Weeks

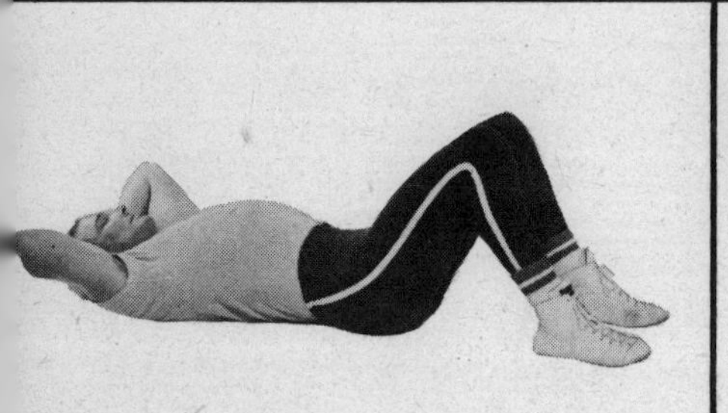

Start Position: Lie flat on floor, knees bent, hands clasped behind head, elbows forward.

***30 seconds at all times**

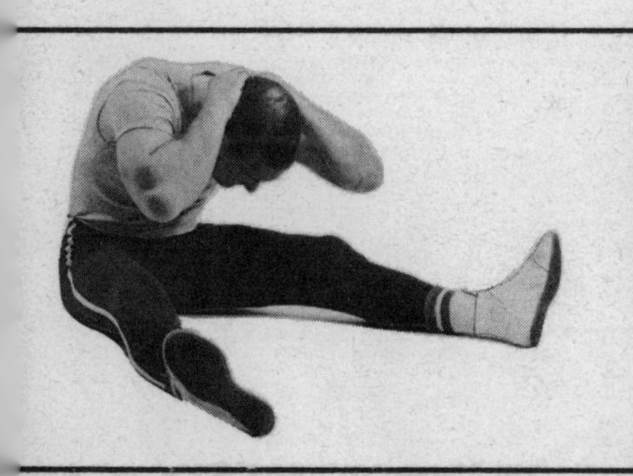

Action-Count 1. Sit up and lean forward until elbows touch knees (try to hold knees straight).

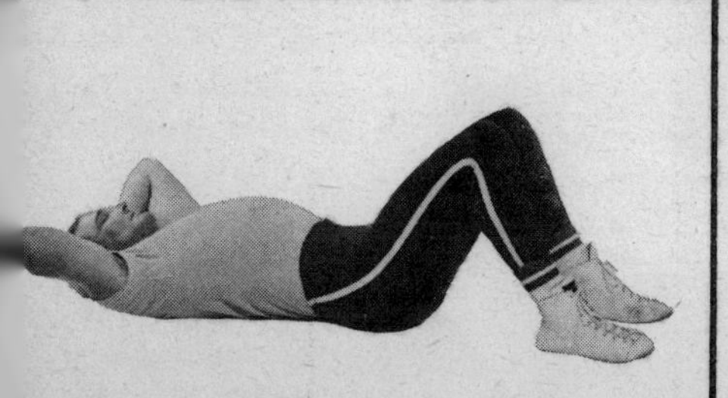

Count 2. Return to start position.

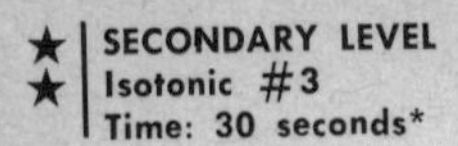

SQUAT THRUSTS

This exercise should be repeated: 14 times, Fourth and Fifth Weeks 15 times, Sixth and Seventh Weeks

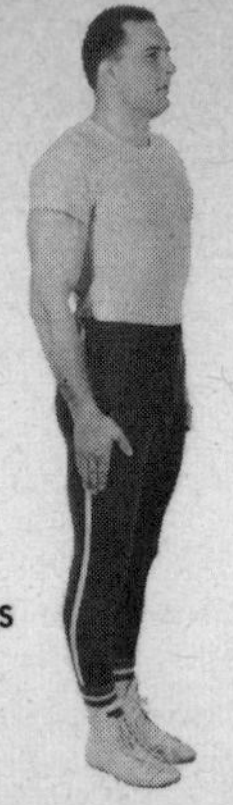

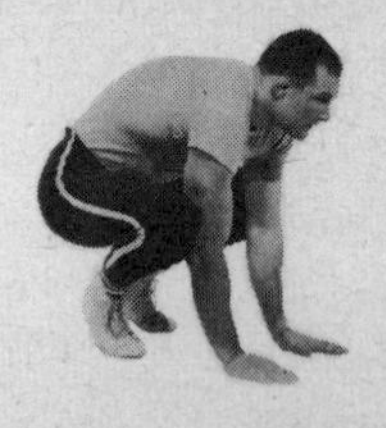

Start Position: Stand erect, legs together, arms at sides.

Action-Count 1. Squat, placing hands flat on floor, elbows straight.

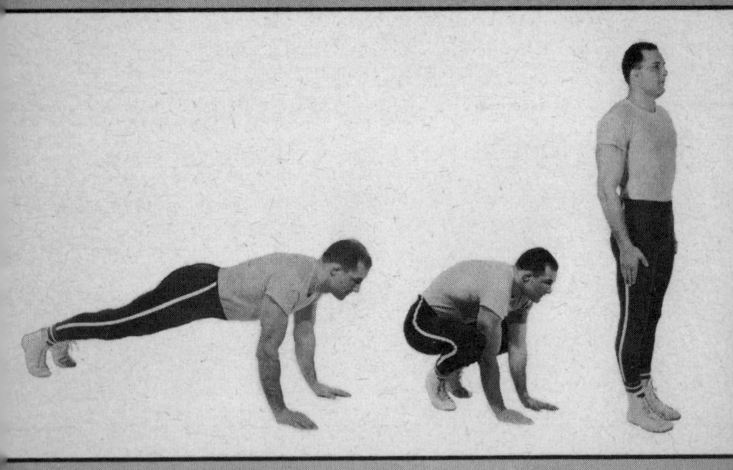

Count 2. Throw both legs straight backwards to extended position.

Count 3. Jump back to squat position as in Count 2.

Count 4. Return to start position.

PUSH-UPS

This exercise should be repeated:
15 times, Fourth and Fifth Weeks
20 times, Sixth and Seventh Weeks
and each two counts equal one repetition.

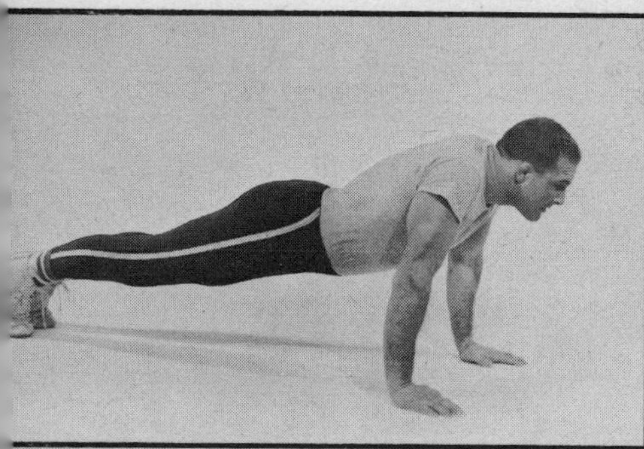

Start Position: Place palms of hands flat on floor in front of you, arms extended, elbows straight, legs and torso extended back in a straight line. Do not bend knees or arch back.

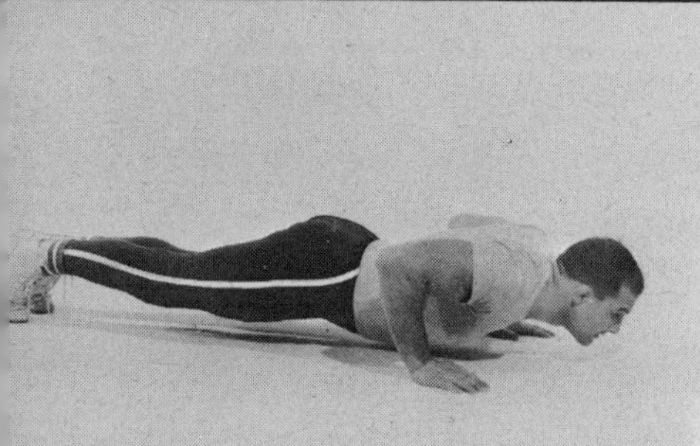

Action-Count 1. Bend elbows lowering chest to, but not touching, floor. Back and legs remain in straight line.

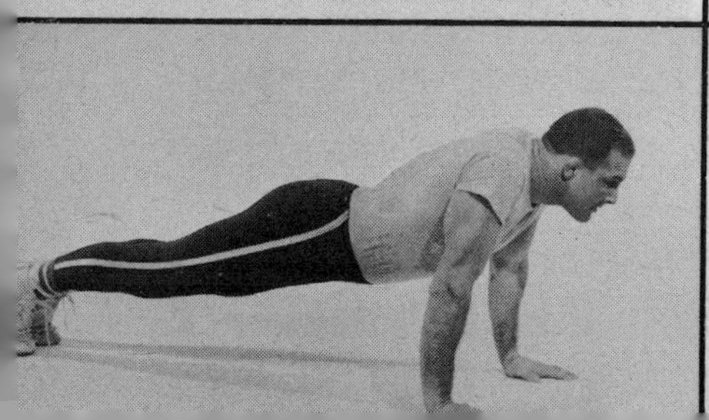

Count 2. Return to start position.

**30 seconds at all times*

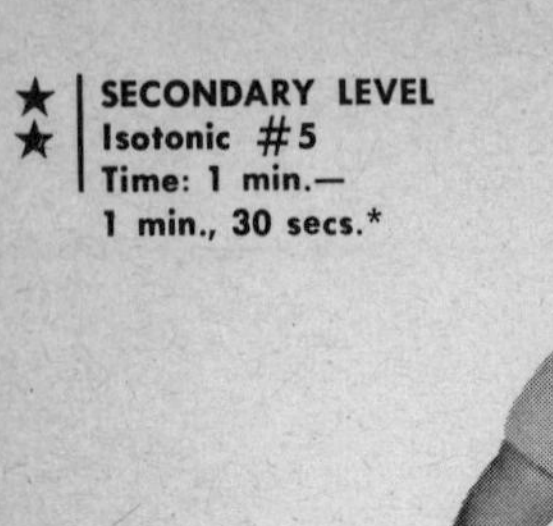

SECONDARY LEVEL
Isotonic #5
Time: 1 min.—
1 min., 30 secs.*

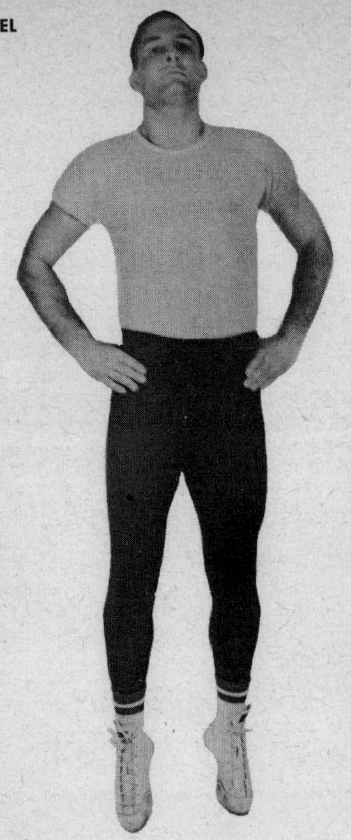

****1 minute, Fourth and Fifth Weeks***
****1 minute, 30 seconds, Sixth and Seventh Weeks***

IMAGINARY ROPE SKIP

This exercise should be repeated:
120 times, Fourth and Fifth Weeks
175 times, Sixth and Seventh Weeks

Hop in place for allotted time, clearing floor with enough height to go over an imaginary rope. (Some exercisers find this easier to do if they turn their wrists while hopping as if rope skipping.) Keep count throughout and time this exercise accurately.

★ ★ ★ PEAK LEVEL

The Isometric-Isotonic Total-Fitness Plan permits the exerciser to go on to the Peak Level *after* the Secondary Level has been completed, for now the isotonic exercises can be done with ease. This should be achieved by the eighth week of the course. This will vary, of course, from person to person, for reasons of age, weight, and general condition at the start of the Plan.

Therefore, if you find it difficult to execute the exercises at this Level in the allotted time, *return to the Secondary Level, Chart II, and stay there for at least an additional week.* Then attempt the Peak Level again, bearing in mind that this is the competitive-athlete level. If this is beyond your needs, merely stay at the Secondary Level, which will keep you trim and fit for as long as you do it.

The differences between this Level and the Secondary Level is that three isotonic exercises are changed and the number of repetitions increased.

★ ★ ★ PEAK LEVEL

CHART I

8th and 9th Weeks

	Exercise	Repetitions	Time in Secs
WARM-UP	1. Stretch and Bend	12	30
	2. Squat and Touch	10	30
	3. Knee Hug	10	30
	4. Twist and Touch	10	45
	5. Seal Bend	10	40
ISOMETRIC	1. Doorway Press	1	10
	2. Lateral Raise	1	10
	3. Knee Pull	1	10
	4. Knee-Press (Interior)	1	10
	5. Knee-Press (Exterior)	1	10
	6. Abdominal Contraction	1	10
	7. Dead Lift	1	10
	8. Under Leg Curl	1	10
	9. Doorway Toe Raise	1	10
	10. Toe Pull	1	10
ISOTONIC	1. Jumping Jack	42	30
	2. Knee Bent Sit-Up	12	30
	3. Squat Thrust	18	30
	4. Push-Ups	34	30
	5. Squat Jump	25	30

CHART II

After 10th Week or for Heavy Athletics

	Exercise	Repetitions	Time in Secs
WARM-UP	1. Stretch and Bend	12	30
	2. Squat and Touch	10	30
	3. Knee Hug	10	30
	4. Twist and Touch	10	45
	5. Seal Bend	10	40
ISOMETRIC	1. Doorway Press	1	10
	2. Lateral Raise	1	10
	3. Knee Pull	1	10
	4. Knee-Press (Interior)	1	10
	5. Knee-Press (Exterior)	1	10
	6. Abdominal Contraction	1	10
	7. Dead Lift	1	10
	8. Under Leg Curl	1	10
	9. Doorway Toe Raise	1	10
	10. Toe Pull	1	10
ISOTONIC	1. Jumping Jack	82	1-min.
	2. Knee Bent Sit-Up	17	45
	3. Squat Thrust	26	45
	4. Push-Ups	40	40
	5. Squat Jump	35	40

BEND AND STRETCH

This exercise should be repeated *12 times.*

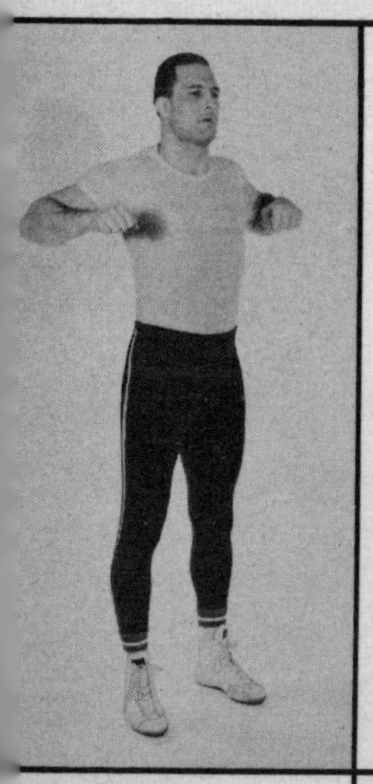

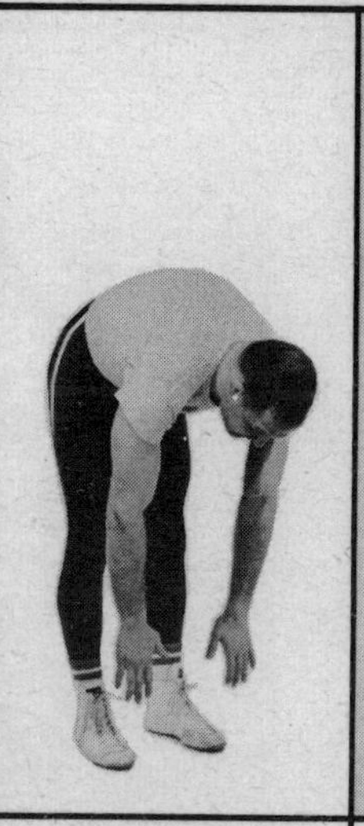

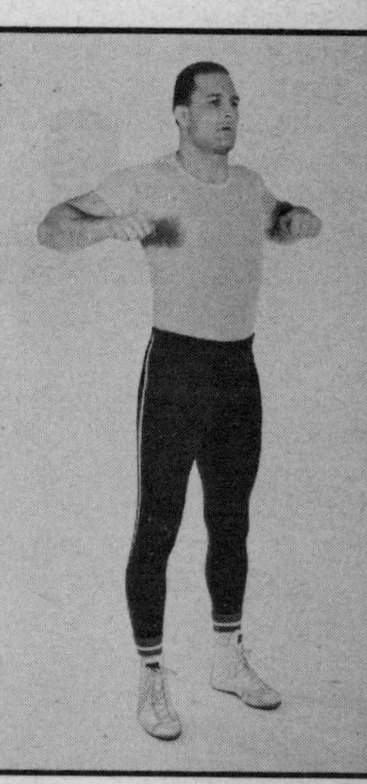

Start position: Stand erect, arms at shoulder level, fists clenched, elbows bent and thrust back as far as possible.

Action-Count 1. Bend forward to floor, with arms hanging down and fingers relaxed. Bend knees slightly and allow head to hang forward.

Count 2. Return to start position.

★ **PEAK LEVEL**
★ **Warm-up #2**
★ **Time: 30 seconds**

SQUAT AND TOUCH

This exercise should be repeated *10 times.*

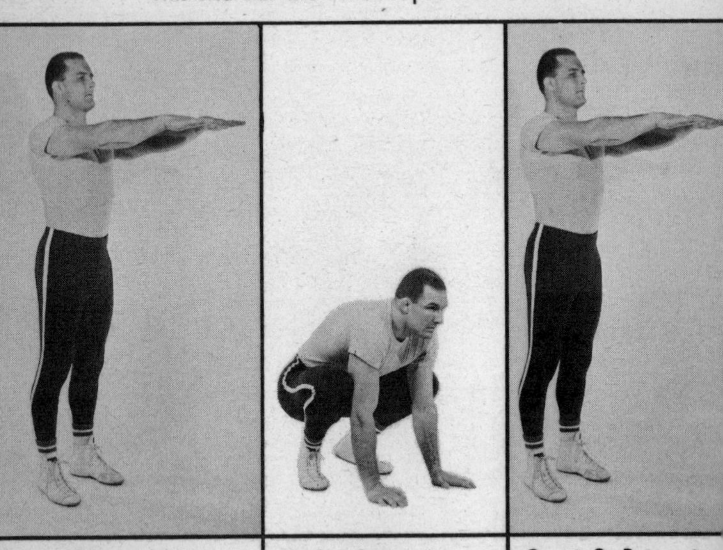

Start position: Stand erect, arms extended to front, palms down, feet about 12 inches apart.

Action-Count 1. Bend knees and squat, touching fingers or palms of hands to floor between knees. Keep head erect and back straight.

Count 2. Return to start position.

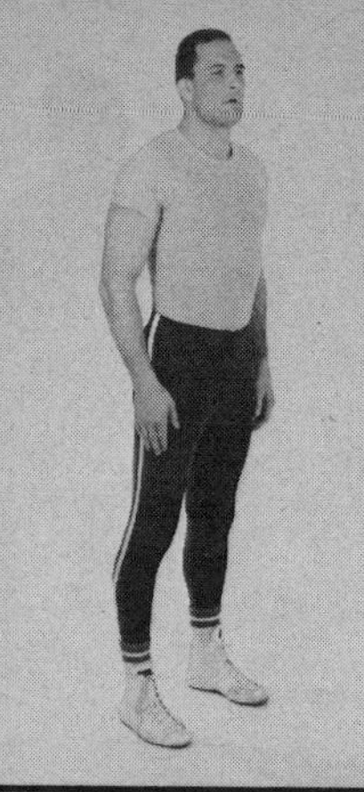

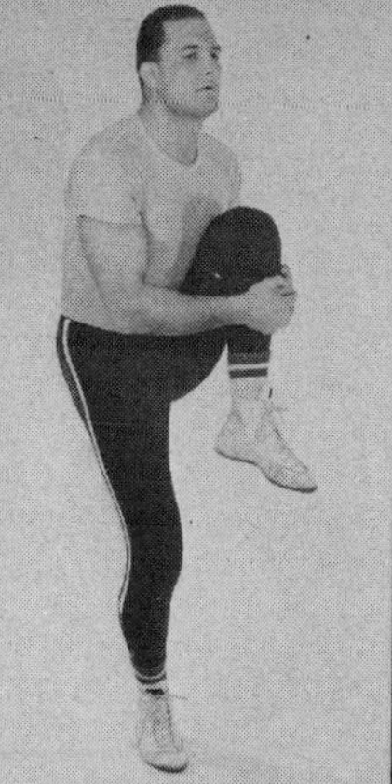

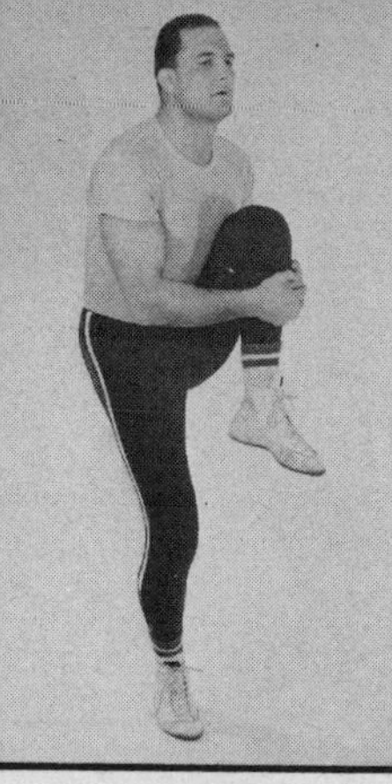

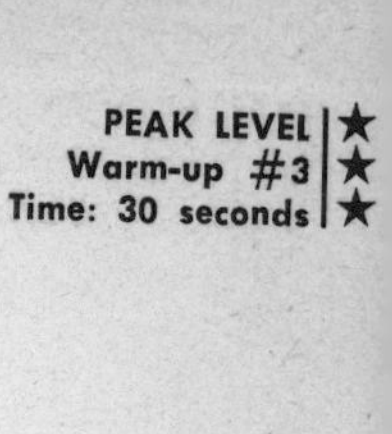

Start Position: Stand erect, back straight, arms at sides.

Action-Count 1. Raise left knee to chest level. Grasp lower leg with both hands and draw leg to chest.

KNEE-HUG

This exercise should be repeated *10 times,* and each repetition represents 4 counts.

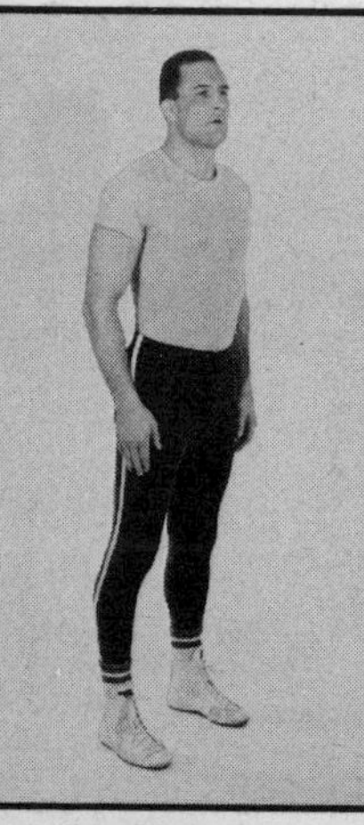

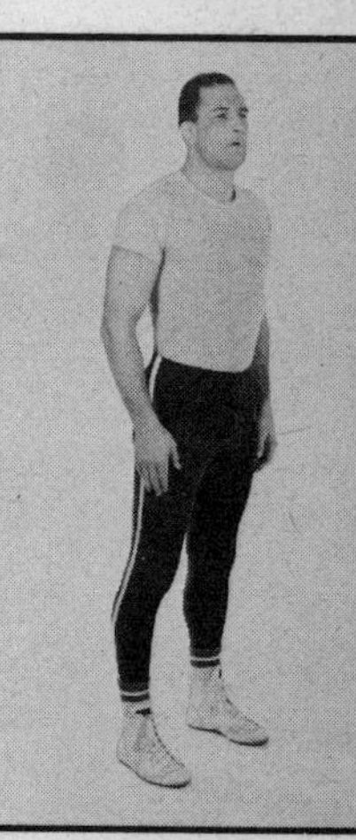

Count 2. Return to start position.

Count 3. Raise right knee to chest as in Count 1.

Count 4. Return to start position.

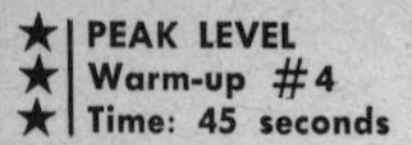

★ PEAK LEVEL
★ Warm-up #4
★ Time: 45 seconds

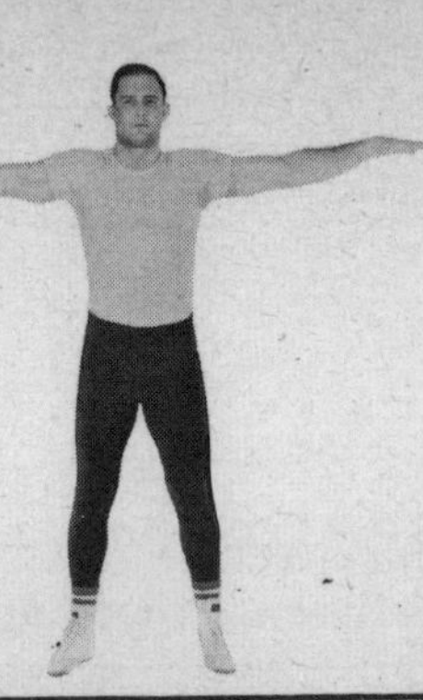

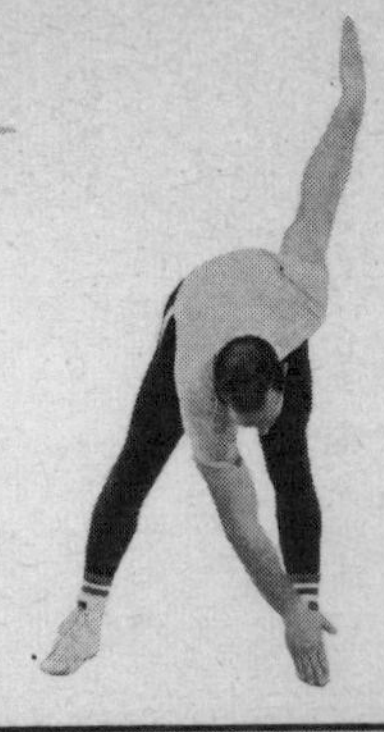

TWIST AND TOUCH

This exercise should be repeated *10 times,* and each repetition represents 4 counts.

Start position: Stand erect, arms extended at sides, palms down, legs apart.

Action-Count 1. Twist to left, touching right fingertips to left toe, extending left arm vertically. (Left knee may be slightly bent.)

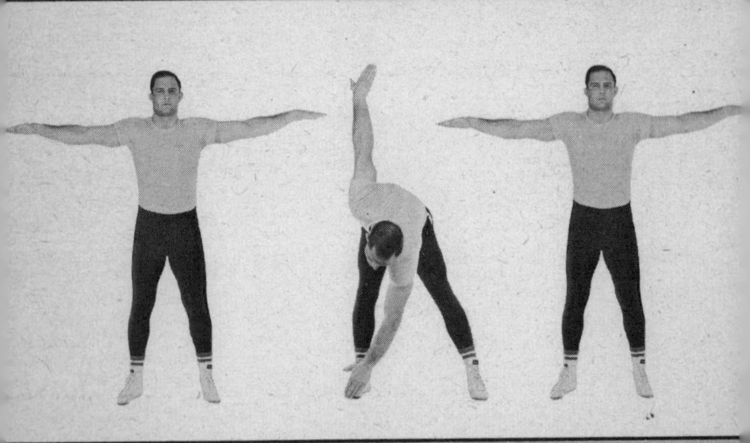

Count 2. Return to start position.

Count 3. Repeat Action-Count 1, but in opposite direction.

Count 4. Return to start position.

SEAL BEND

This exercise should be repeated *10 times.*

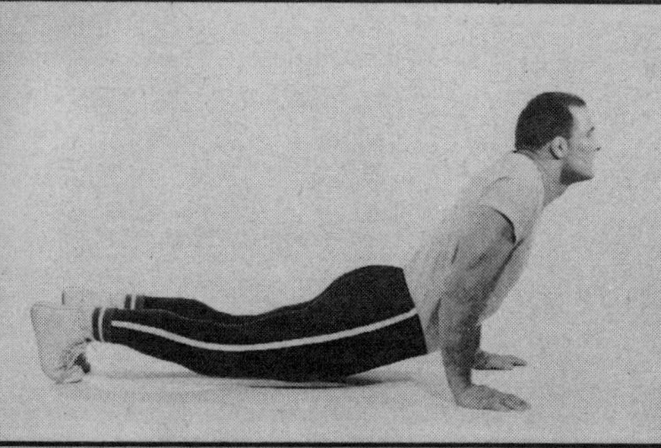

Start position: On floor, extend legs straight back and together, arms straight from shoulder to floor, back arched so hips almost touch floor.

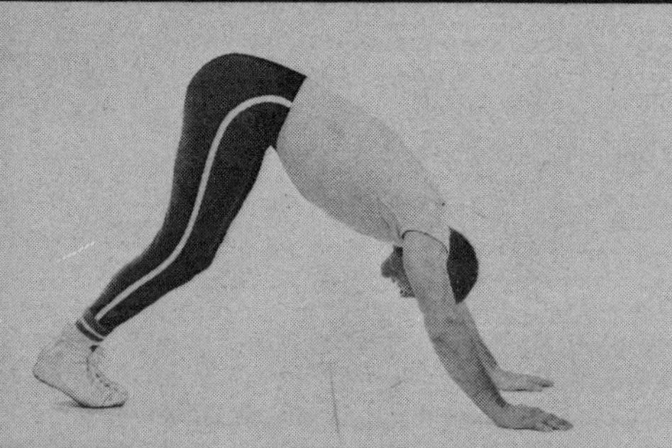

Action-Count 1. Raise hips as high as possible, at the same time push head down between arms.

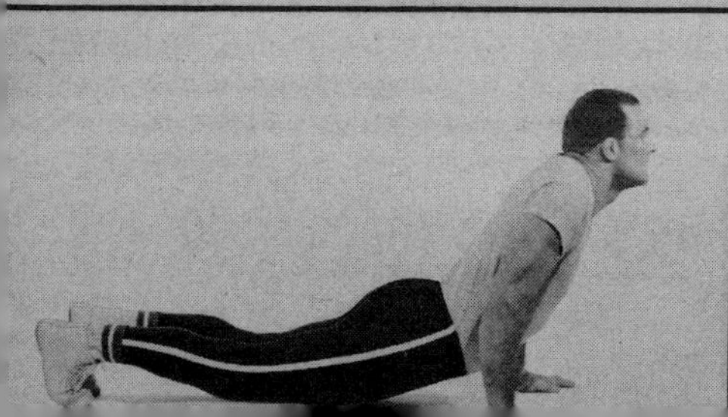

Count 2. Return to start position.

★ ★ ★ PEAK LEVEL

ISOMETRIC PERIOD

The isometric contractions at Peak Level are the same as those described in the Secondary Level, except that now *the degree of intensity of your maximum effort in each contraction will be raised* from what it was when you started the program. If you wish to measure your strength by lifting a weight, you will discover, on completion of the Peak Level, how much more you can lift than when you started the plan.

The nature of these contractions are such that they encompass the various areas of the body that should be strengthened in a total-fitness program.

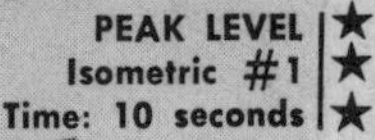

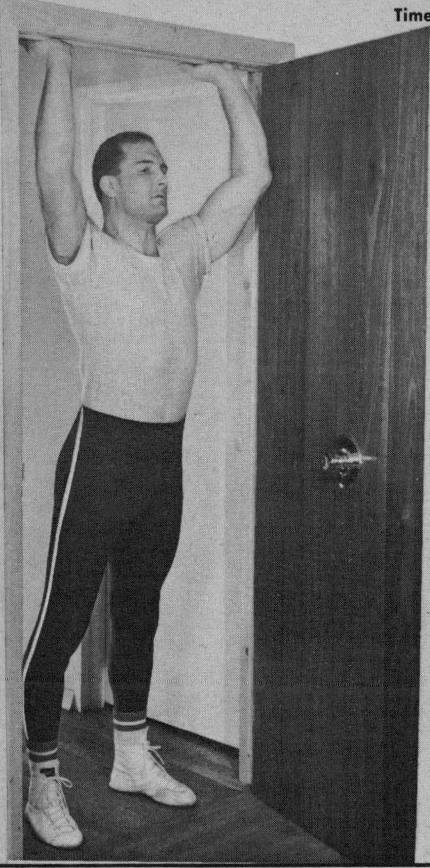

DOORWAY PRESS

Position: Stand erect in doorway. Place palms of hands on top of doorway, arms bent halfway. (If you do not reach the top of door stand on some books or ther solid base until you do.)

Contraction: Inhale. Using arms and back, press upward with palms of hands against top of door. Increase pressure for 4 seconds until maximum effort is reached. Hold maximum effort for 6 seconds.

Relax and exhale.

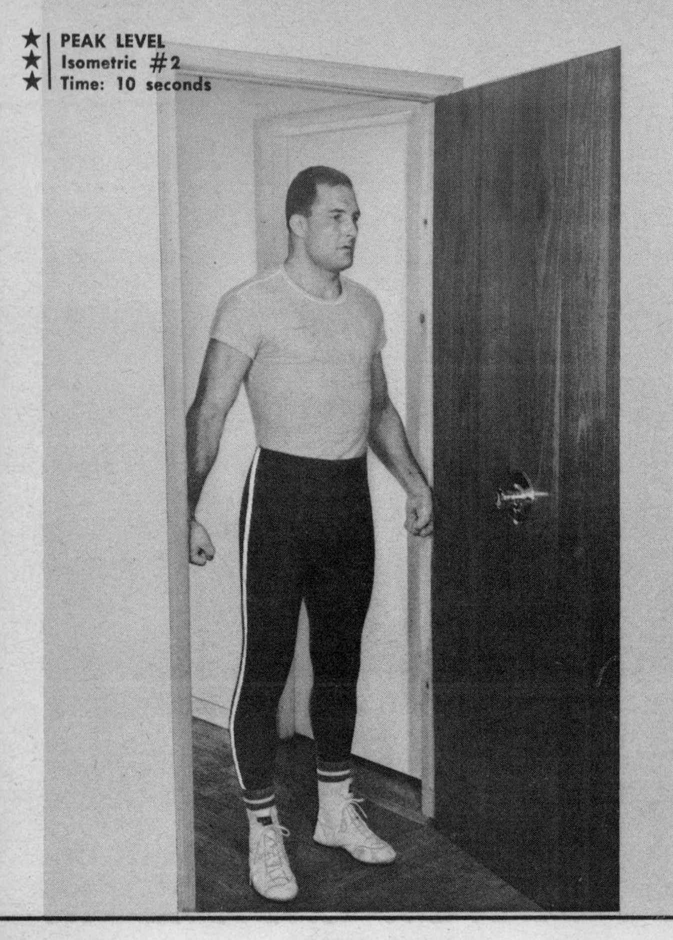

LATERAL RAISE

Position: Stand erect in doorway. Place backs of hands against sides of door, touching on both sides.

Contraction: Inhale. Attempt to raise both arms simultaneously upward and sideward. Increase pressure for 4 seconds until maximum effort is reached. Hold maximum effort for 6 seconds.

Relax and exhale.

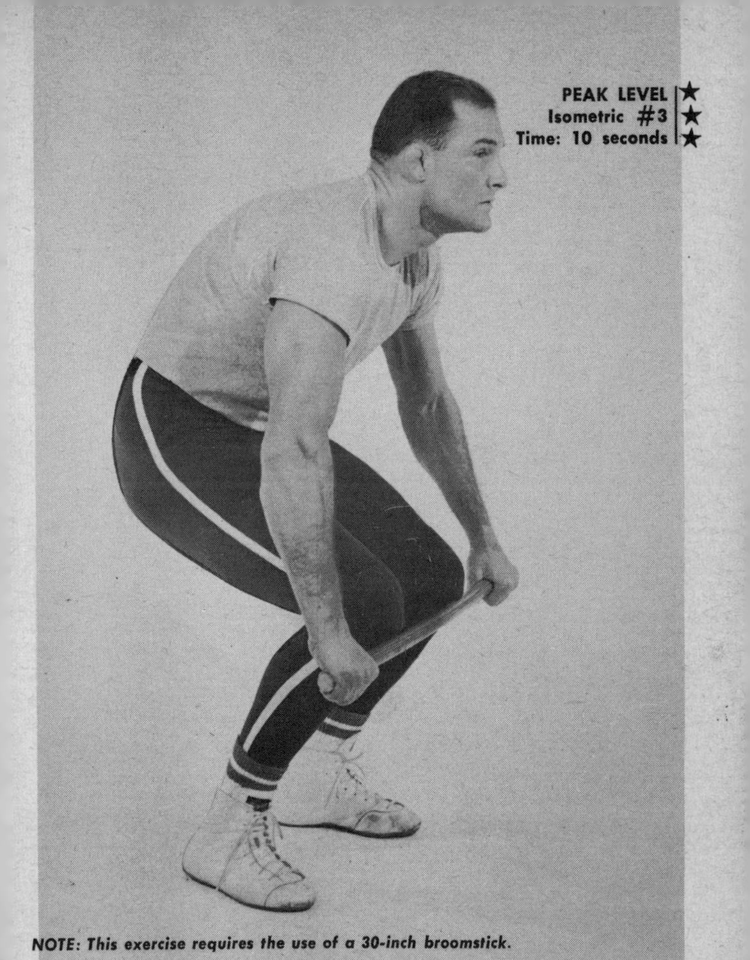

NOTE: This exercise requires the use of a 30-inch broomstick.

KNEE PULL

Position: Semi-squat. Place broomstick in front of knees. (Place knees as close to ends of stick as possible, allowing enough of stick to extend at either end for firm grasp.)

Contraction: Inhale. Pull backward and upward, with back and arms against broomstick. Increase pressure for 4 seconds. Hold maximum effort for 6 seconds.

Relax and exhale.

★ PEAK LEVEL
★ Isometric #4
★ Time: 10 seconds

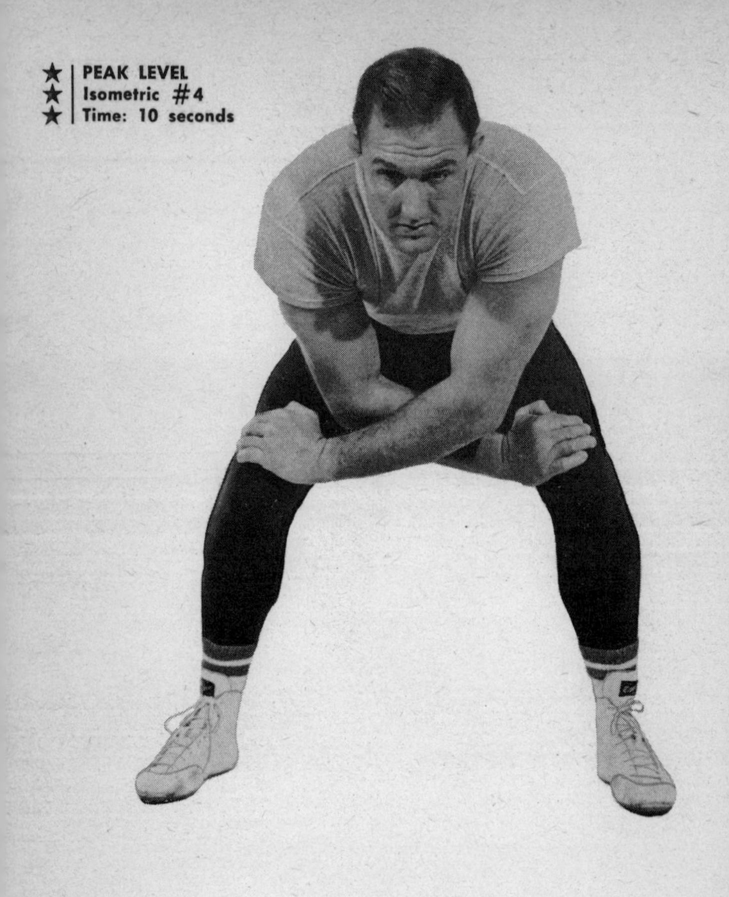

KNEE-PRESS (INTERIOR)

Position: Semi-squat forward, cross arms and place palms of hands against *insides* of opposite knees.

Contraction: Inhale. Press palms outward against insides of knees and simultaneously try to force knees together. Increase effort for 4 seconds until maximum effort is reached. Hold maximum effort for 6 seconds.

Relax and exhale.

PEAK LEVEL ★
Isometric #5 ★
Time: 10 seconds ★

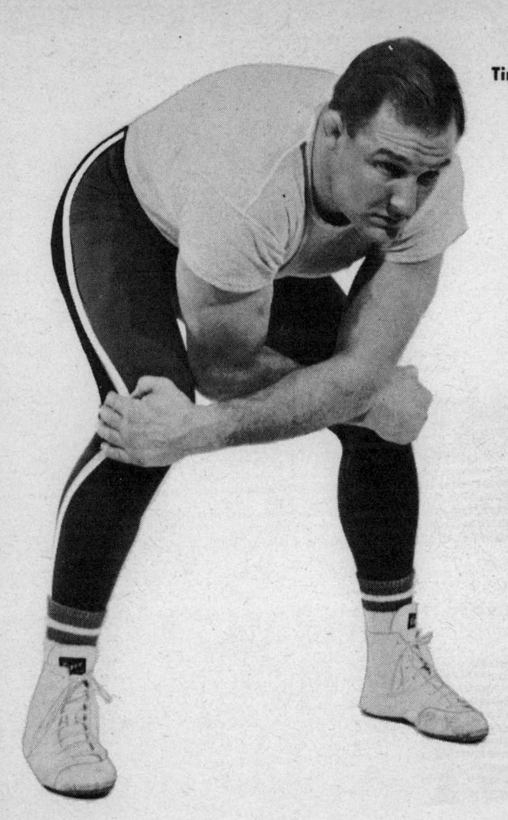

KNEE PRESS (EXTERIOR)

Position: Semi-squat forward. Cross arms and grasp outside of opposite knees.

Contraction: Inhale. Attempt to pull knees together with hands, at the same time force knees apart with legs. Increase effort for 4 seconds and hold maximum effort for 6 seconds.

Relax and exhale.

★ PEAK LEVEL
★ Isometric #6
★ Time: 10 seconds

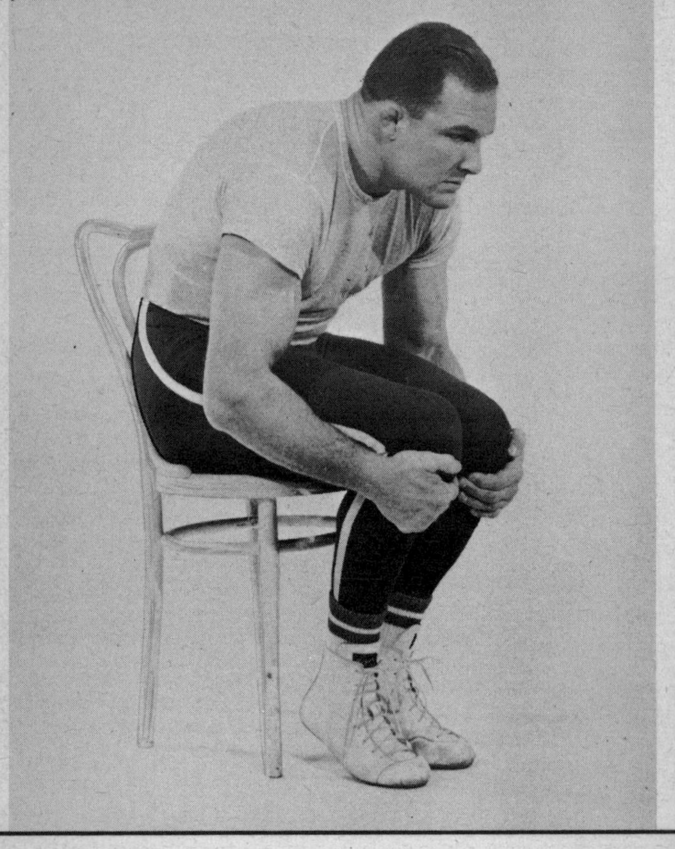

ABDOMINAL CONTRACTION AND HEEL PRESS

Position: Sit in chair, legs together, heels raised off floor. Lean forward and grasp both knees with hands.

Contraction: Inhale. Tense stomach, attempt to force heels to floor. At the same time, pull back on knees so that heels cannot be lowered. Increase force of action for 4 seconds. Hold maximum effort for 6 seconds.

Relax and exhale.

PEAK LEVEL ★
Isometric #7 ★
Time: 10 seconds ★

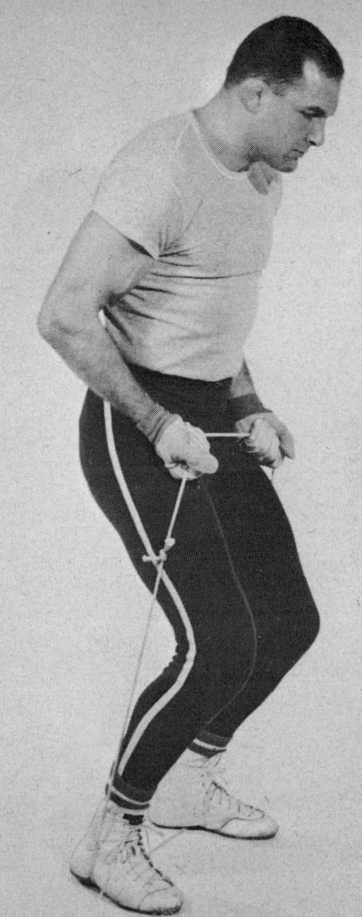

NOTE: This exercise requires the use of a rope (or clothesline) as before.

DEAD LIFT

Position: Stand with both feet within loop. Grasp loop at sides with both hands, palms up. Assume semi-squat position with back straight. Take up slack in loop by winding excess rope around hands.

Contraction: Inhale. Using legs and back, attempt to come erect against resistance of loop. Increase pressure for 4 seconds. Hold maximum effort for 6 seconds.
Relax and exhale.

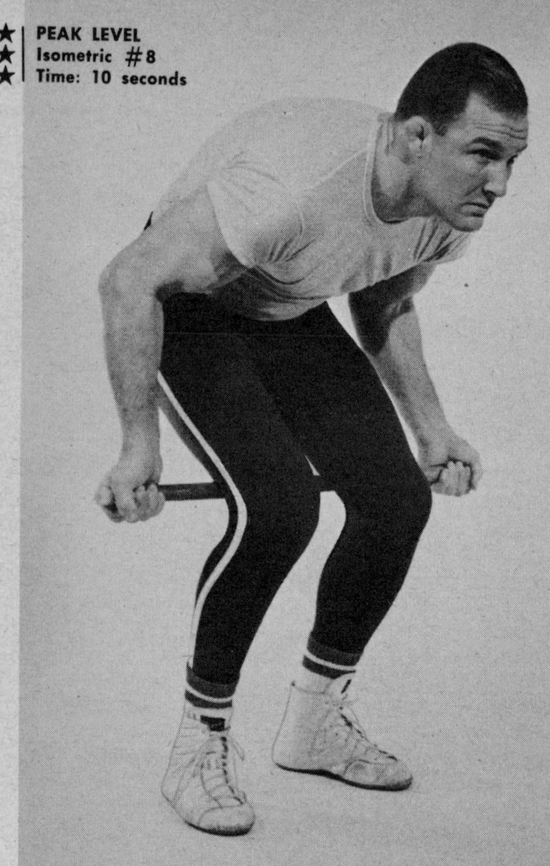

Note: This exercise requires the use of a 30-inch broomstick.

UNDER LEG CURL

Position: Place stick behind knees, grasping both ends with palms up. Assume semi-squat position.

Contraction: Inhale. Curl arms forward and upward, increasing pressure for 4 seconds. Hold maximum effort for 6 seconds.

Relax and exhale.

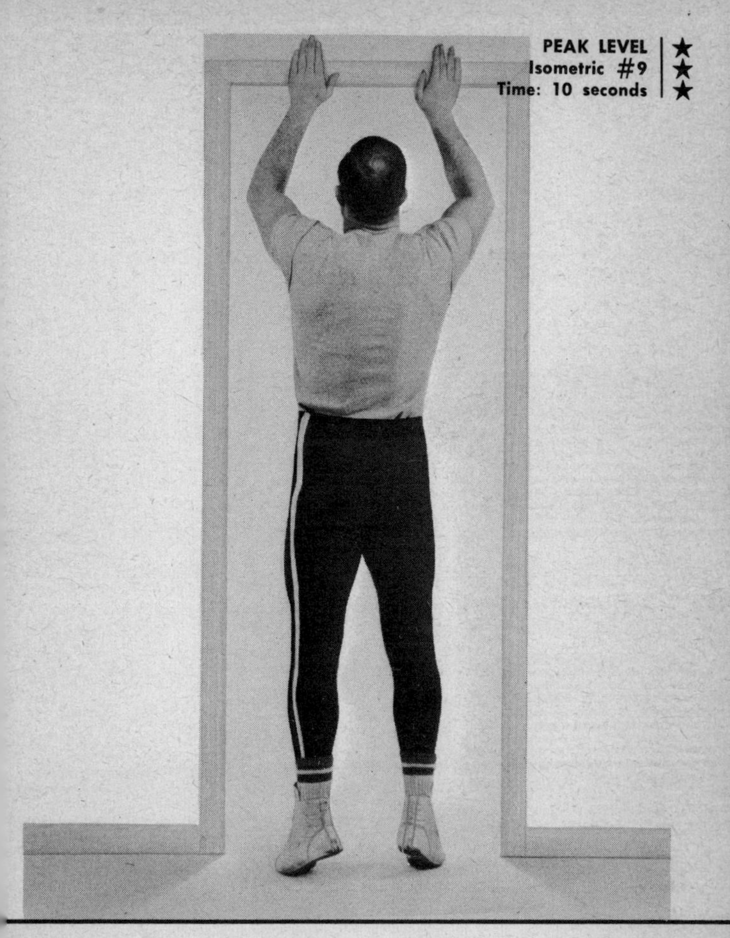

DOORWAY TOE RAISE

Position: Stand in doorway with palms of hands against top of doorway, arms extended. Raise up on toes until heels are off floor about one inch.

Contraction: Inhale. Push against top of doorway with arms straight so heels go back to floor, at the same time push back with calves of legs so that heels stay up. Increase pressure for 4 seconds. Hold maximum effort for 6 seconds.

Relax and exhale.

★ PEAK LEVEL
★ Isometric #10
★ Time: 10 seconds

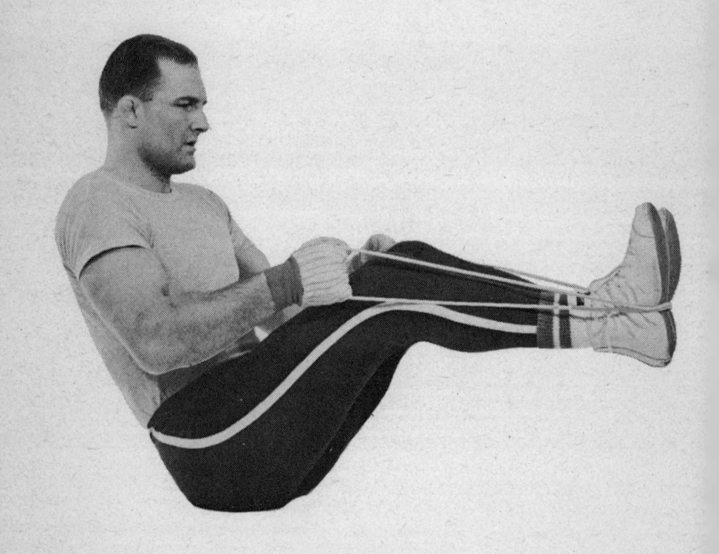

***NOTE:* This exercise requires the use of rope (or clothesline) as before.**

TOE PULL

Position: Sit on floor, both sides of loop under feet, grasping ends of loop with both hands. Lift legs off floor so lower leg is parallel with floor.

Contraction: Inhale. Attempt to extend both legs while restraining with arms. Increase pressure for 4 seconds until maximum effort is attained. Hold maximum effort for 6 seconds.

Relax and exhale.

★ ★ ★ PEAK LEVEL

ISOTONIC PERIOD

This period is designed to extend the efficiency of the cardiovascular system so that it will respond favorably to vigorous exertion. An athlete who can perform these exercises in the times allotted will be of championship caliber.

The exercises selected will neither interfere with nor impede skills needed for specialized activities like putting the shot or fencing, for instance. They are general in scope and thus can only help improve total performance.

★ PEAK LEVEL
★ Isotonic #1
★ Time: 30 secs.—1 min.*

JUMPING JACK

This exercise should be repeated:
42 times, Eighth and Ninth Weeks
82 times, Tenth Week

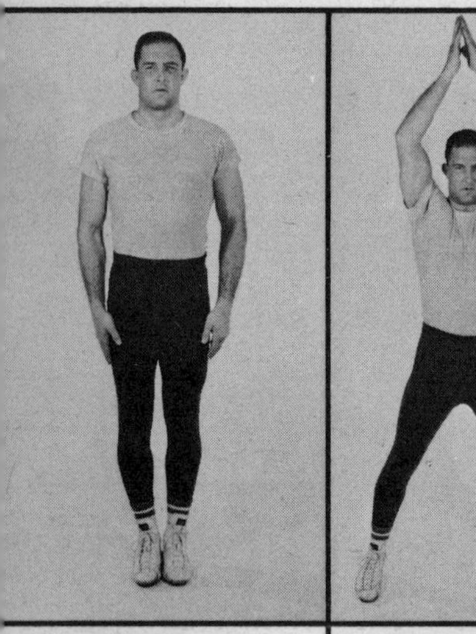

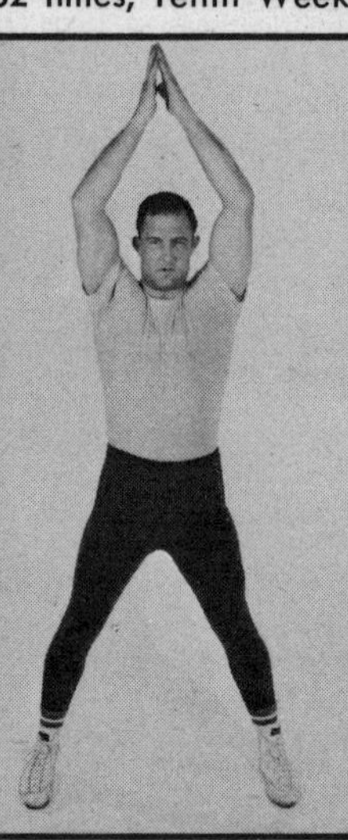

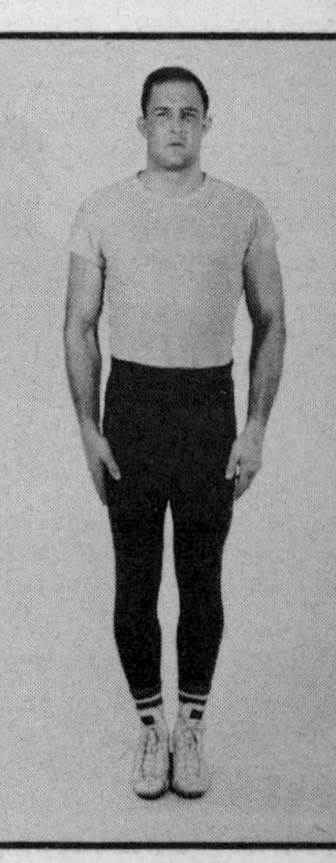

Start Position: Stand erect hands at side, legs together.

Action-Count 1. Jump to legs apart, simultaneously raising arms sidewards overhead, elbows straight, and clap hands.

Count 2. Jump back to start position.

**30 seconds, Eighth and Ninth Weeks*
**1 minute, Tenth Week*

KNEE-BENT SIT-UP

This exercise should be repeated:
12 times, Eighth and Ninth Weeks
17 times, Tenth Week

PEAK LEVEL ★★★
Isotonic #2
Time: 30-45 seconds*

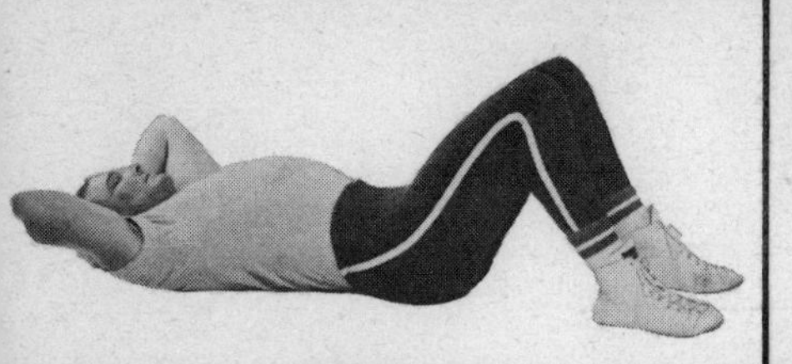

Start Position: Lie flat on floor, hands clasped behind neck, knees bent.

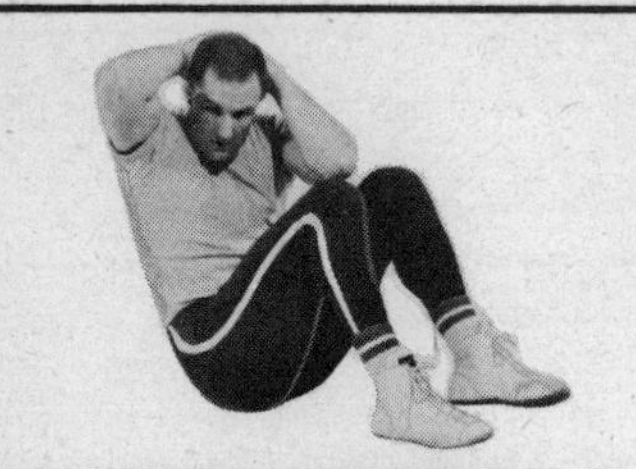

Action-Count 1. Sit up, touching left elbow to right knee.

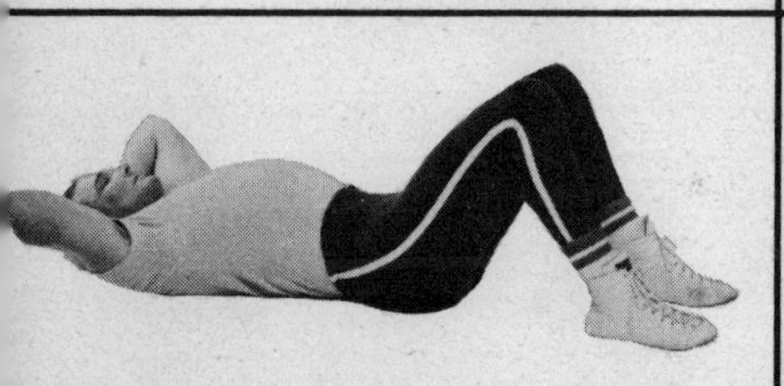

Count 2. Return to start position.

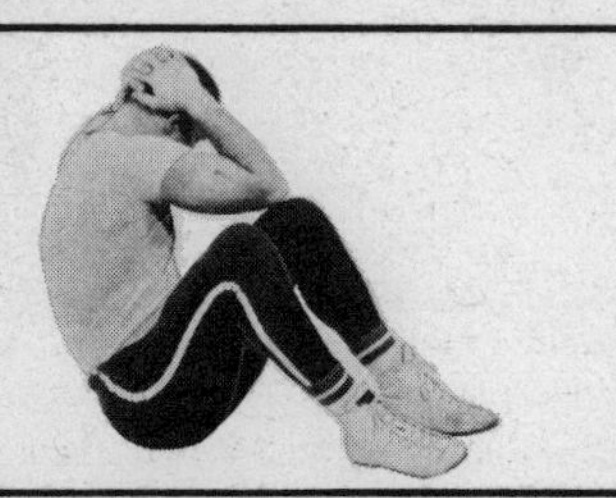

Count 3. Sit up, touching right elbow to left knee.

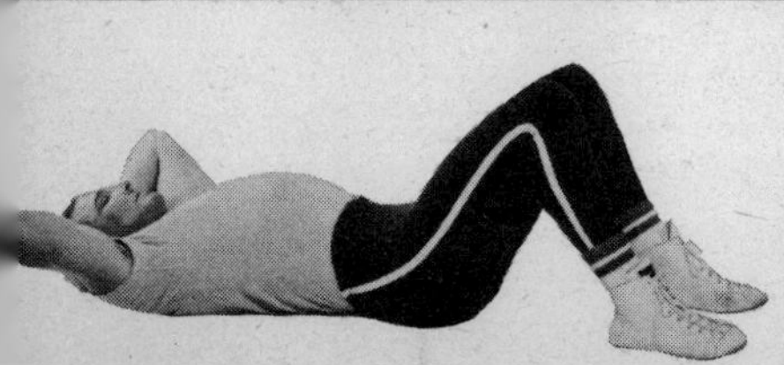

Count 4. Return to start position.

****30 seconds, Eighth and Ninth Weeks*
45 seconds, Tenth Week*

★ PEAK LEVEL
★ Isotonic #3
★ Time: 30-45 seconds*

SQUAT THRUST

This exercise should be repeated: 18 times, Eighth and Ninth Weeks 26 times, After Tenth Week or for heavy athletics

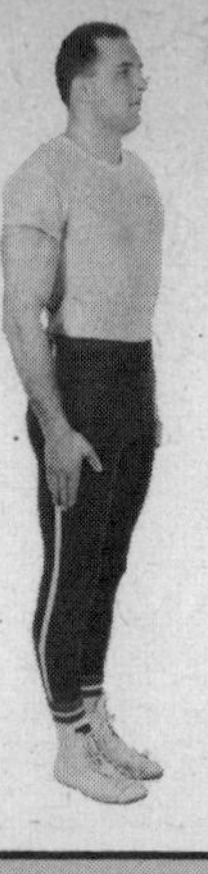

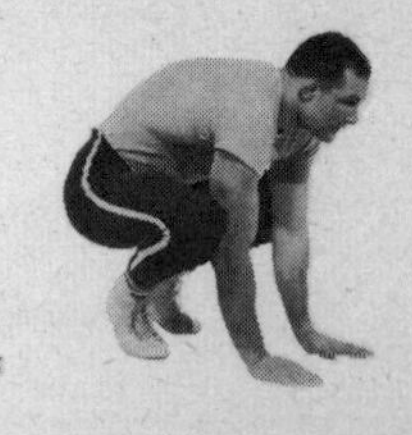

Start Position: Stand erect, legs together, arms at sides.

Action-Count 1. Squat, placing hands flat on floor, elbows straight.

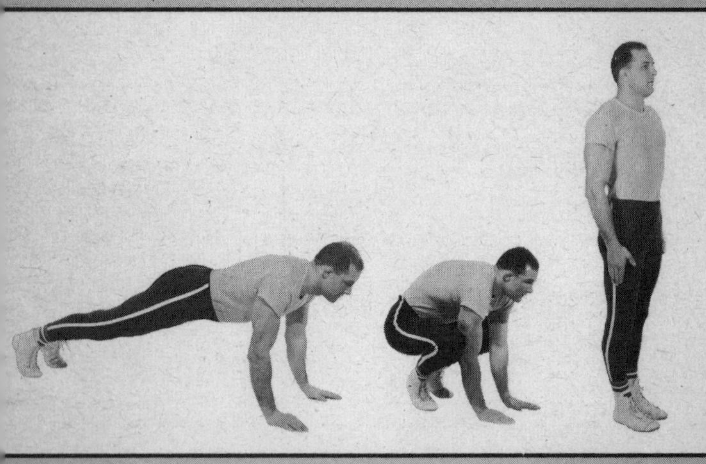

Count 2. Throw both legs straight backwards to extended position.

Count 3. Jump back to squat position as in Count 2.

Count 4. Return to start position.

**30 seconds, Eighth and Ninth Weeks*
**45 seconds, Tenth Week*

PUSH-UPS FROM CHAIR

This exercise should be repeated:
34 times, Eighth and Ninth Weeks
40 times, Tenth Week

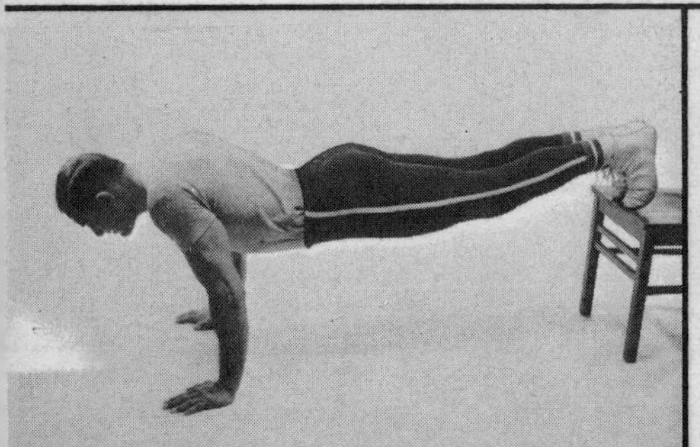

Start Position: Place toes on chair, extend body and legs forward in a straight line, arms extended in front of chest, elbows straight, palms of hands flat on floor.

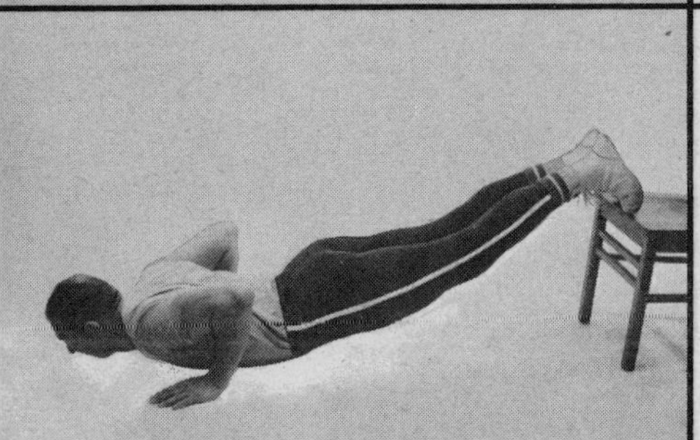

Action-Count 1. Bend elbows so that chest drops to, but does not touch, floor. Body and legs remain rigid.

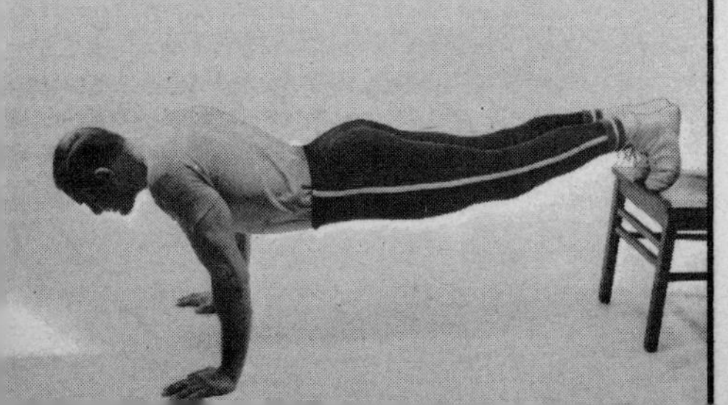

Count 2. Return to start position.

****30 seconds, Eighth and Ninth Weeks***
****40 seconds, Tenth Week***

★ | **PEAK LEVEL**
★ | **Isotonic #5**
★ | **Time: 30-40 seconds***

SQUAT JUMP

This exercise should be repeated:
25 times, Eighth and Ninth Weeks
35 times, Tenth Week
and *each jump counts 1 full repetition.*

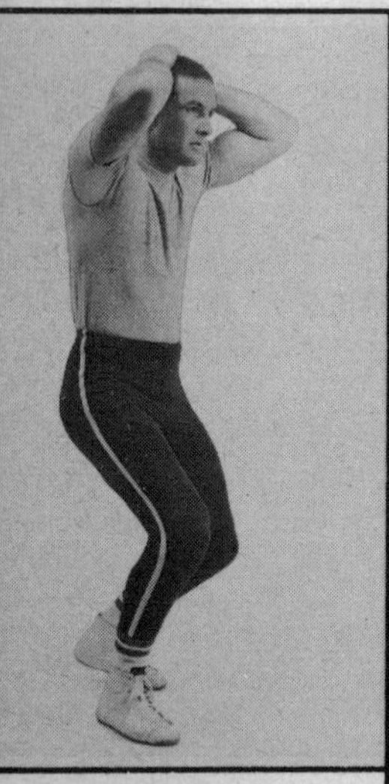

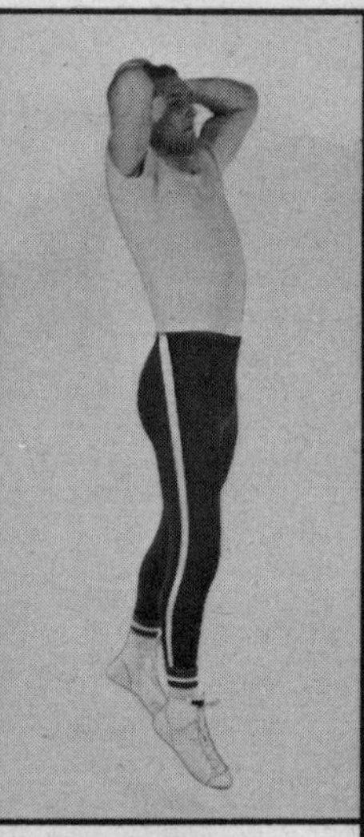

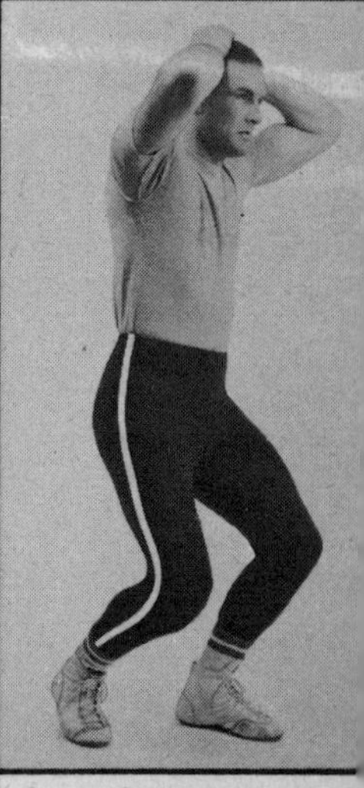

Start Position: Place clasped hands on top of head, half-squat with right foot forward, left knee facing down, feet about 8 inches apart.

Action-Count 1. Jump straight up, high enough to change position of legs in mid-air so left foot is forward, and you land in a semi-squat position.

Count 2. Jump from squat, bringing right foot forward to mid-air and return to original start position.

****30 seconds, Eighth and Ninth Weeks***
****40 seconds, Tenth Week***

ALTERNATE ISOMETRIC PERIOD

Whenever it is necessary to skip your regular isometric-isotonic session, the following series of contractions should be done as a substitute workout.

These can be done at your desk, in your automobile, in the morning, or before going to bed. They need no warm-up period and can be done while you are fully clothed.

The contractions should be memorized and done in the sequence shown. If done *once each daily,* these will maintain your current fitness level until you can get back to your regular program.

Although the entire workout takes less than two minutes, your strength and general condition will improve even if no other exercises are done.

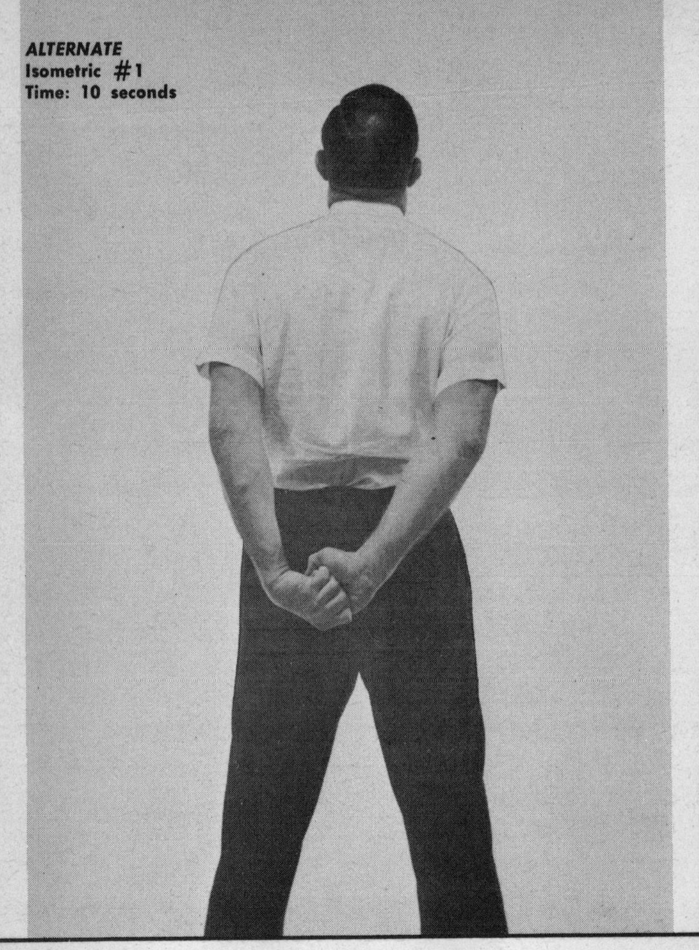

BACK ARM PULL

Position: Stand or sit erect. Hook fingers behind your back in the *Isometric Grip*. Straighten arms backward as far as they will go.

Contraction: Inhale. Keep arms stiff. Try to pull arms apart. Maintaining grip (so that no movement is possible) increase pressure for 4 seconds. Hold maximum effort for 6 seconds.

Relax and exhale.

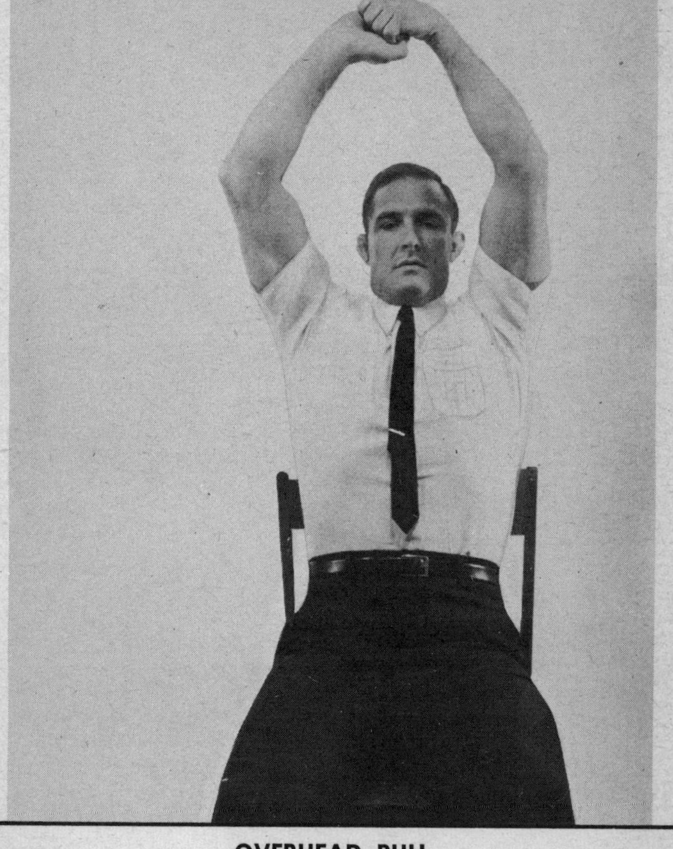

OVERHEAD PULL

Position: Stand or sit erect. Join hands overhead in an interlocking grip.

Contraction: Inhale. Pull arms outward against grip, increasing effort for 4 seconds. Hold maximum effort for 6 seconds.

Relax and exhale.

ALTERNATE
Isometric #3
Time: 10 seconds

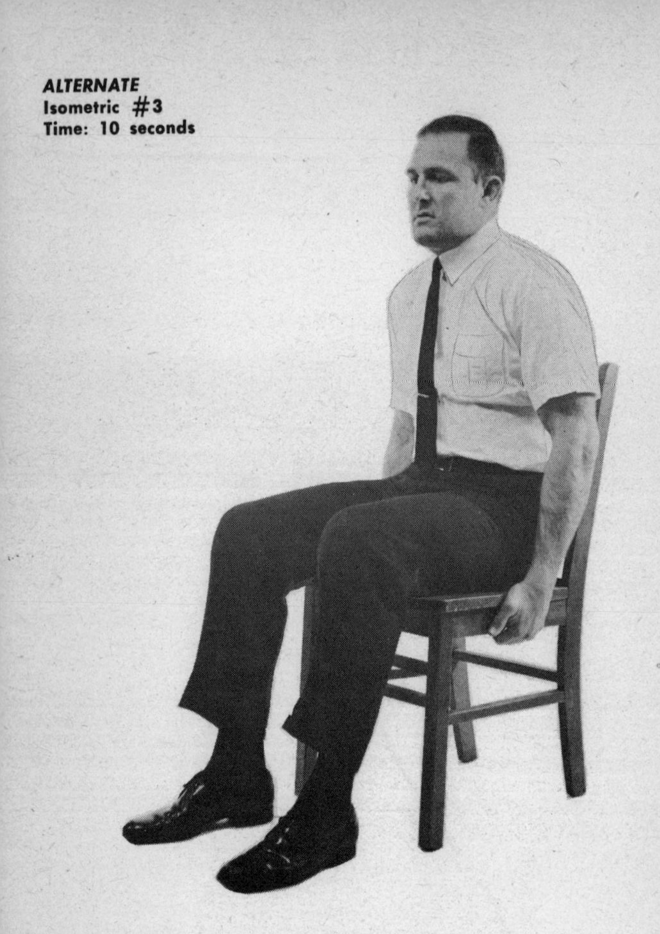

CHAIR LIFT

Position: Sit erect in chair. Grasp seat of chair on both sides with hands.

Contraction: Inhale. Attempt to lift yourself *and* seat of chair off the floor. Increase pressure for 4 seconds. Hold maximum effort for 6 seconds.

Relax and exhale.

ALTERNATE
Isometric #4
Time: 10 seconds

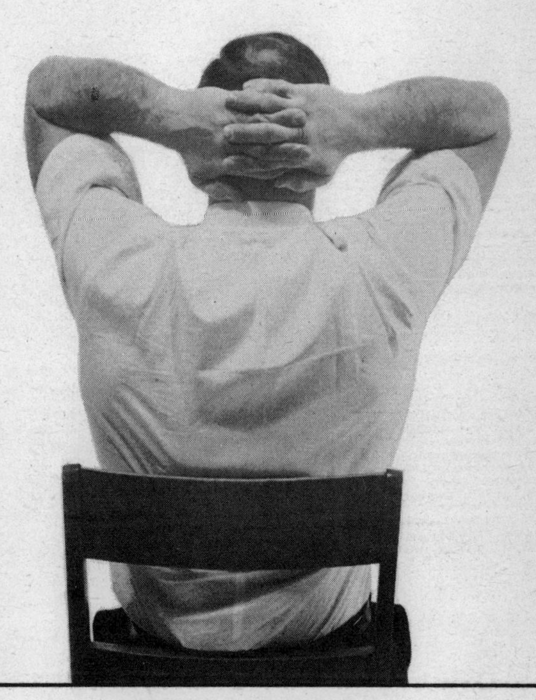

BEHIND NECK PULL

Position: Standing erect, (or seated) place hands behind head, elbows bent forward, fingers interlaced.

Contraction: Inhale. Push against back of head with hands, pushing back with head. Increase pressure for 4 seconds. Hold maximum effort for 6 seconds.

Relax and exhale.

ALTERNATE
Isometric #5
Time: 10 seconds

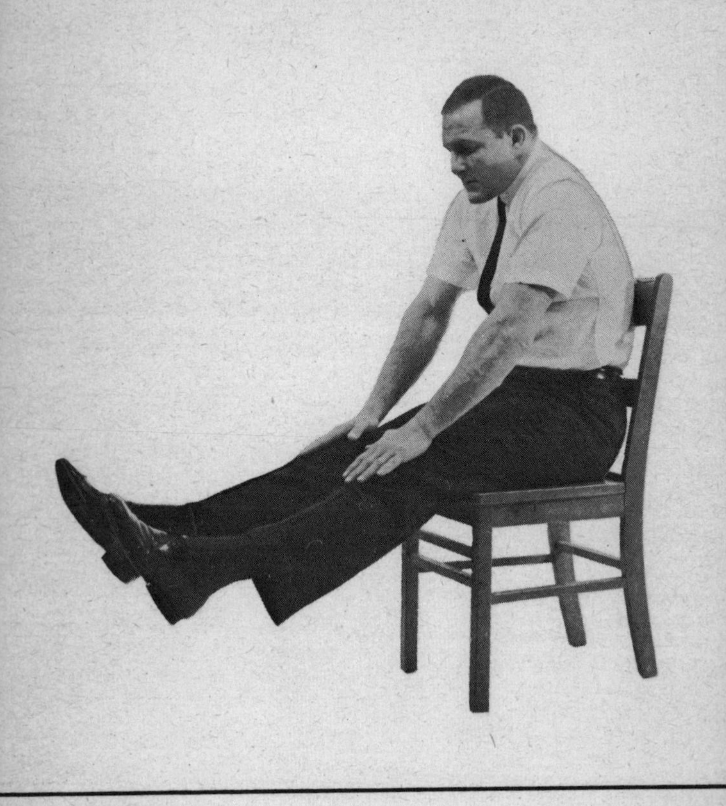

FORWARD LEAN

Position: Sit in chair. Extend legs with knees straight in front, feet together and about a foot from floor. Place hands upon knees, keeping arms straight.

Contraction: Inhale. Press hands down on knees, keeping knees in place at same time. Increase pressure for 4 seconds. Hold maximum effort for 6 seconds.

Relax and exhale.

ALTERNATE
Isometrics #6, #7
Time: 10 seconds each

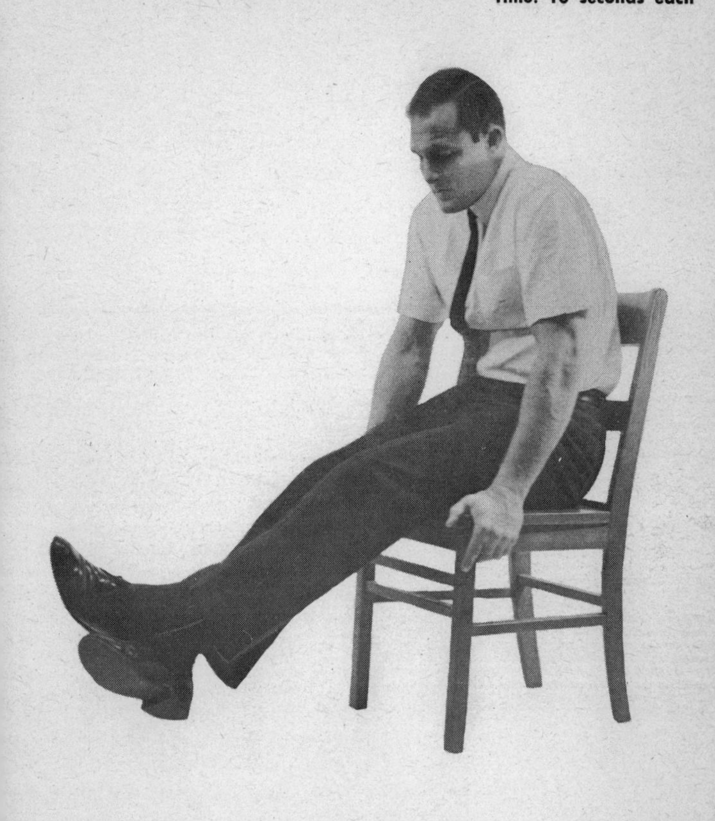

ANKLE PRESS

Position: Seated erect in chair, cross ankles with right ankle beneath, and pressing against, back of left ankle.

Contraction: Inhale. Force left foot back against right ankle, at the same time push right foot forward against left ankle. Increase pressure for 4 seconds and hold maximum effort for 6 seconds.

Relax and exhale.

Repeat contraction, placing left ankle beneath right ankle.

ISOMETRIC-ISOTONIC TOTAL-FITNESS PLAN FOR WOMEN

Isometric contractions in a fitness plan for women are especially effective: They can be applied to specific areas and result in quick firming and strengthening. Too, isometrics are one of the finest forms of exercise for return to normal after childbirth, or in post-operative cases, but in these instances *it is imperative that the contractions be embarked upon only under medical supervision.*

The fact that improvement occurs rapidly with isometric contractions also holds true for the healthy individual. Women who have used isometrics have had amazingly rapid, beneficial results. Flabby tissue firms up in less than two weeks and energy and well-being improve at the same time. As with any other type of exercise, isometrics alone will not cause an appreciable loss of weight. But together with a reducing diet, this can help take pounds off your body and give you a more youthful appearance.

Women who wish to participate in the isometric-isotonic total-fitness plan, must first learn the technique of applying maximum effort in an isometric contraction.

●

First, place your wrist watch or a clock with a sweep-second hand before you so that you can easily read the dial.

●

Extend both arms in front of you with the palms of your hands touching. Now inhale a three-quarter breath and hold it.

●

Watching the seconds' hand of the clock, begin to exert pressure by pushing one palm against the other. The pressure should be equalized between the arms so that there is a deadlock at all times and *no movement.* Remember, *in an isometric contraction there is* no *movement.*

•

For three seconds, increase the force with which you press your hands together. By the third second you should be straining with such force that you could not possibly increase the pressure, no matter how hard you tried.

•

At this point, a quivering should take place in your arms.

•

You have now reached the point of *maximum effort*—a very important aspect of the isometric contraction. Do not relax or let up on the pressure, but hold this effort for four seconds more, or a total of seven seconds from the time that you started the contraction. At the end of the seven-second effort, relax and exhale.

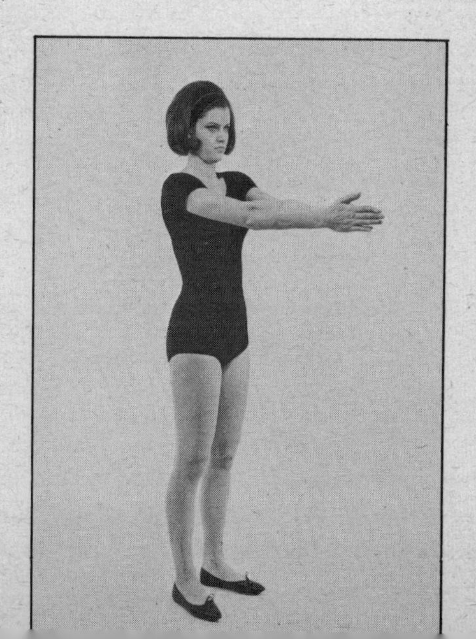

Practice holding your breath during each contraction and exerting maximum effort. As soon as you master the technique, which should take but a few moments, you are ready to begin.

•

Note: Do not exercise before you are fully awake in the morning, or immediately after you have eaten.

•

The isometric-isotonic total-fitness plan for women consists of two parts. These may be done at all levels of condition and at all ages to develop and maintain a good figure, to improve appearance or to supply renewed vitality.

The first part, or *isotonic* period, consists of six exercises that involve movements that will burn up calories, give tone to your musculature, and healthfully invigorate your heart and blood vessels. It is an essential warm-up procedure to the contractions that follow.

The second part, or *isometric* period, will firm flabby tissue and shorten sagging muscles. While it will increase strength and vitality, it will *not result in unsightly bulging muscle.*

The total program takes about ten minutes a day and should produce results in one week. There is no need to increase the *amount* of exercise as your condition improves, for the basic feature of isometrics is that the intensity of the contractions automatically becomes greater as the level of your fitness goes up.

TOTAL FITNESS CHART FOR WOMEN—I

First and Second Weeks

	Exercise	Repetitions	Time in Secs
WARM-UP AND ISOTONIC	1. Bend and Stretch	10	20
	2. Knee-Hug	8	30
	3. Sit and Lean	9	30
	4. Knee Push-Up	12	25
	5. Half-Squat	12	25
	6. Leg Raise	12	30
ISOMETRIC	1. Parade Rest	1	7
	2. Palm Press	1	7
	3. Knee Press	1	7
	4. Front Pull	1	7
	5. Overhead Pull	1	7
	6. Back Stretch and Pull	1	7
	7. Thigh Push	1	7
	8. Calf Raise	1	7

TOTAL FITNESS CHART FOR WOMEN—II

Third Week and Thereafter

	Exercise	Repetitions	Time in Secs
WARM-UP AND ISOTONIC	1. Bend and Stretch	15	30
	2. Knee-Hug	10	30
	3. Sit and Lean	12	30
	4. Knee Push-Up	15	25
	5. Half Squat	15	30
	6. Leg Raise	15	30
ISOMETRIC	1. Parade Rest	1	7
	2. Palm Press	1	7
	3. Knee Press	1	7
	4. Front Pull	1	7
	5. Overhead Pull	1	7
	6. Back Pull	1	7
	7. Thigh Push	1	7
	8. Calf Raise	1	7

ISOTONIC PERIOD FOR WOMEN

The following six exercises should be done daily and can be done by women of all ages. The exercises should be done as the first part of your workout. They will serve to burn calories, tone up your circulatory system and act as a preliminary warm-up before the isometric period.

You will notice that the number of repetitions increases after the first two weeks of the plan. You need not go any further than the number of repetitions called for in the third week of the plan. The energy build-up that occurs as you become more fit will be used later in the isometric period.

FOR WOMEN
Isotonic #1
Time: 20 seconds

BEND AND STRETCH

This exercise should be repeated *10 times.*

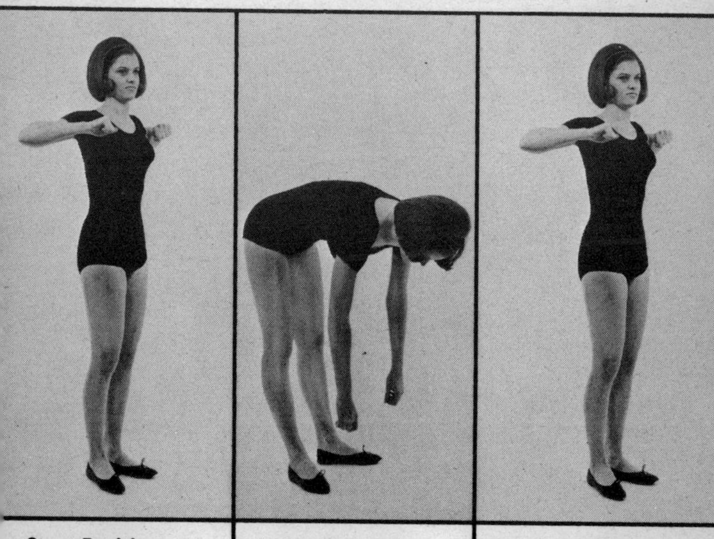

Start Position: Stand erect, arms at shoulder level, fists clenched, elbows bent and thrust back as far as possible.	**Action-Count 1.** Bend forward to floor with arms and fingers relaxed. Bend knees slightly and allow head to hang forward.	**Count 2.** Return to start position.

FOR WOMEN
Isotonic #2
Time: 30 seconds

KNEE-HUG

This exercise should be repeated *8 times.*

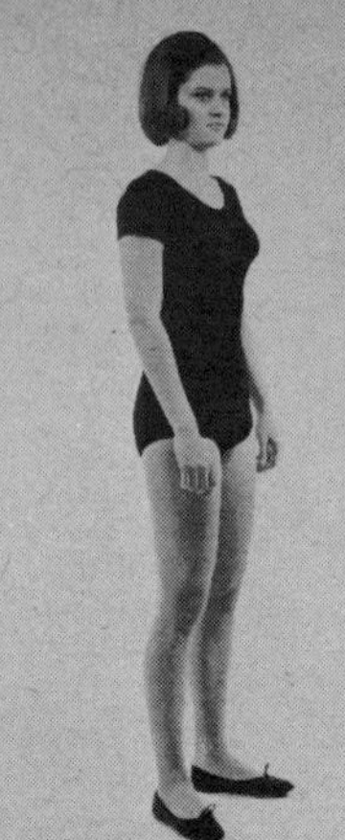

Start Position: Stand erect, back straight, arms at sides.

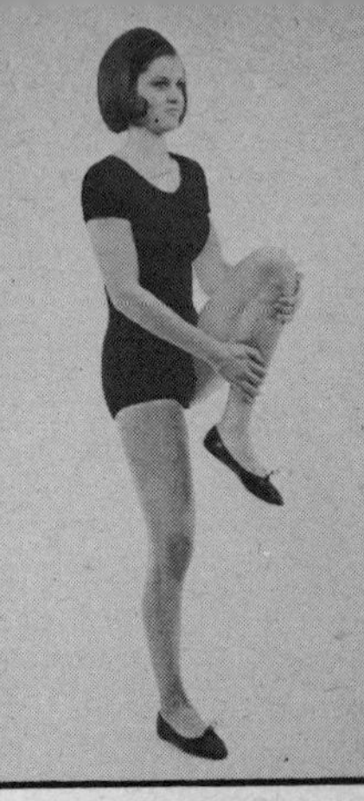

Action-Count 1. Raise left knee to chest level. Grasp lower leg with both hands and draw leg to chest.

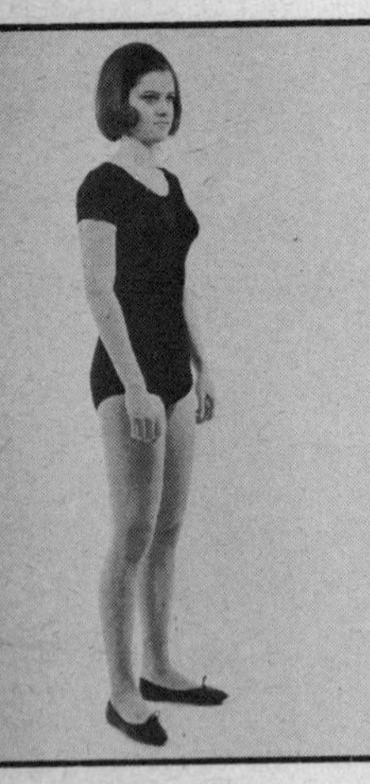

Count 2. Return to start position.

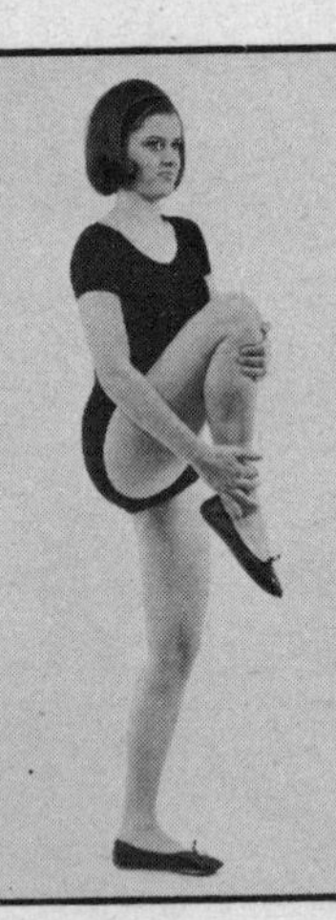

Count 3. Raise right knee to chest as in Count 1.

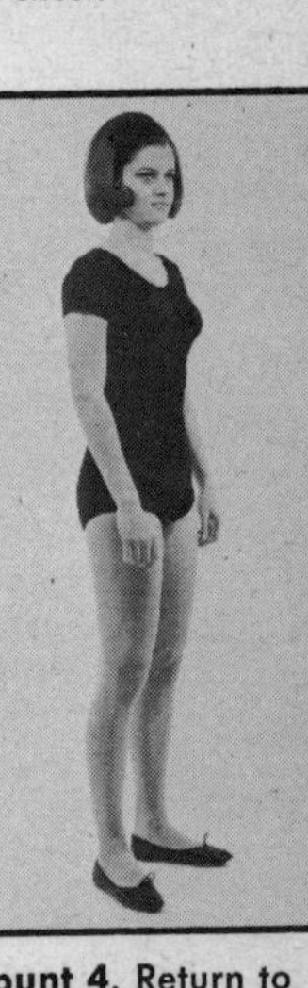

Count 4. Return to start position.

SIT AND LEAN

This exercise should be repeated 9 *times.*

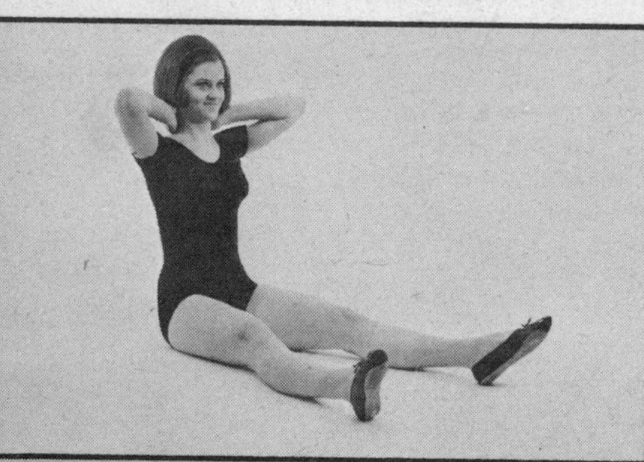

Start Position: Sit on floor, back erect, legs straight and apart. Clasp hands behind neck, elbows pointed out.

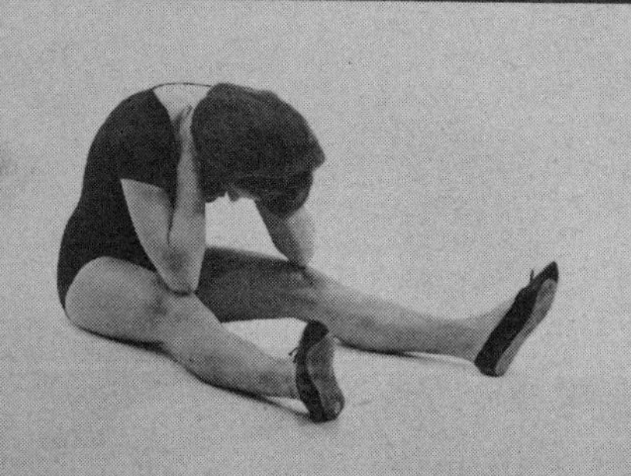

Action-Count 1. Lean forward and try to touch elbows to knees. Keep knees as straight as possible.

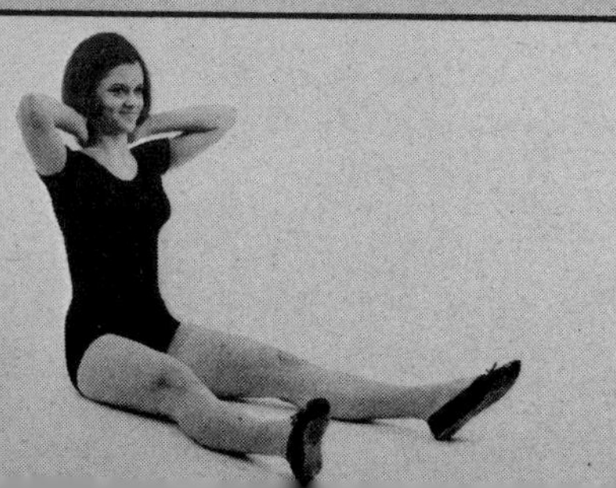

Count 2. Return to start position.

FOR WOMEN
Isotonic #4
Time: 25 seconds

KNEE PUSH-UP

This exercise should be repeated *12 times.*

Start Position: Lie prone on floor, elbows bent, hands flat on floor at chest level.

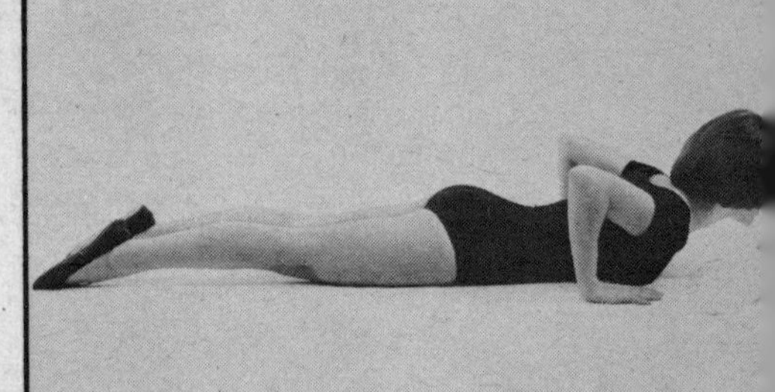

Action-Count 1. Push chest from floor by extending arms to elbow-straight position. Knees are bent and remain on floor as torso is raised.

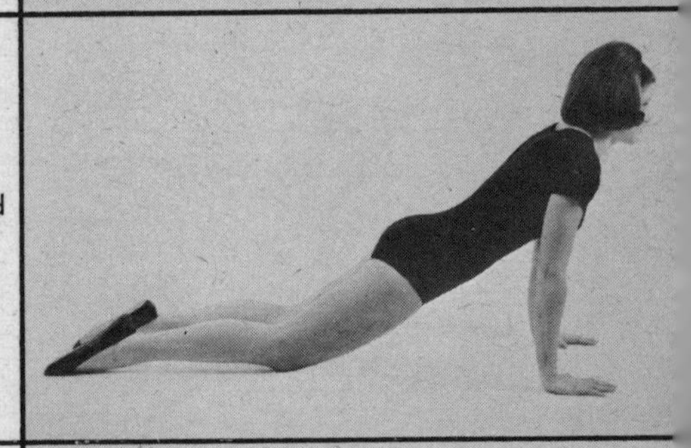

Count 2. Return to start position.

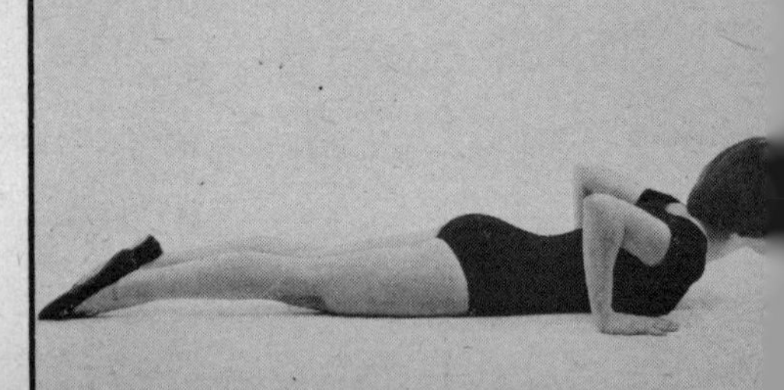

HALF-SQUAT ARMS FORWARD

This exercise should be repeated *12 times.*

(Note: To maintain balance, fix eyes on a stationary object as you go through this exercise.)

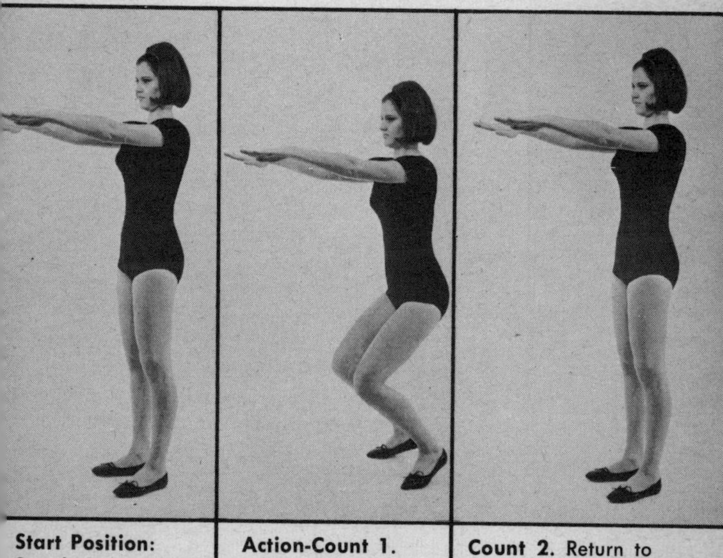

Start Position: Stand erect, arms extended forward, palms facing down.	**Action-Count 1.** Half squat, keeping back straight.	**Count 2.** Return to start position.

FOR WOMEN
Isotonic #6
Time: 30 seconds

LEG RAISE

This exercise should be repeated *12 time*

Start Position: Lie flat on floor, arms at sides, legs together.

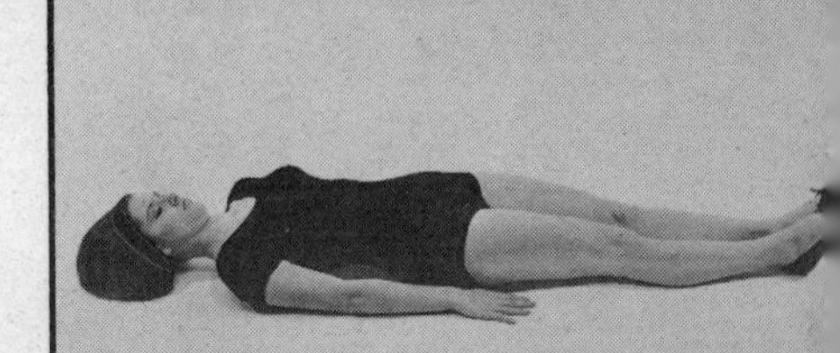

Action-Count 1. Raise legs about 12 inches off floor, toes pointed, knees straight.

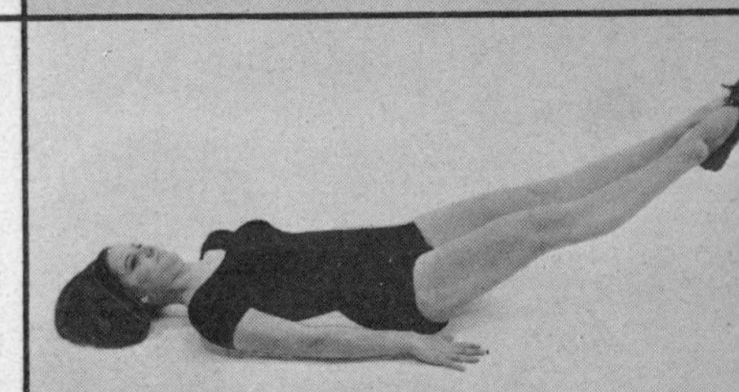

Count 2. Spread legs apart 36 inches or as far as possible, knees straight. (Note: Push down on floor with palms of hands as legs are lifted.)

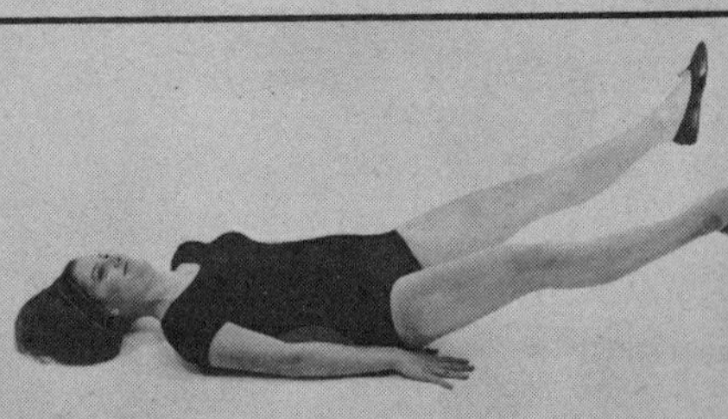

Count 3. Return to legs together position as in Count 1.

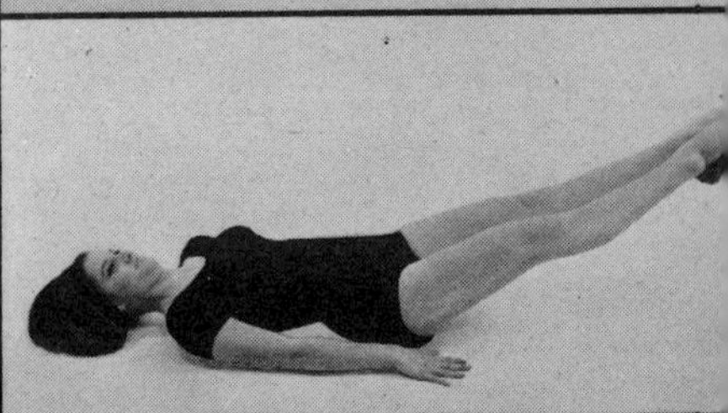

Count 4. Lower legs to floor as in start position.

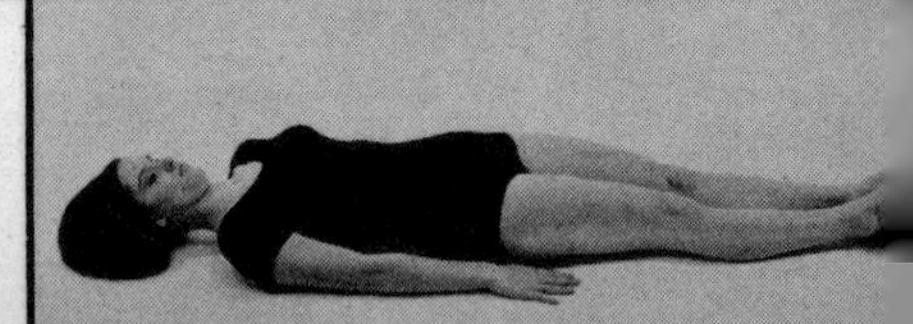

ISOMETRIC PERIOD FOR WOMEN

The following contractions are recommended for women of all ages. They should be done daily, as directed, one minute after the *isotonic* warm-up period.

In the exercises where you are to use the rope loop, tie the ends of a piece of clothesline together to form a loop. If pulling proves uncomfortable, wear a pair of gloves or place a handkerchief between your hand and the rope.

Each exercise in this section for women is to be done *ONLY ONCE.*

FOR WOMEN
Isometric #1
Time: 7 seconds

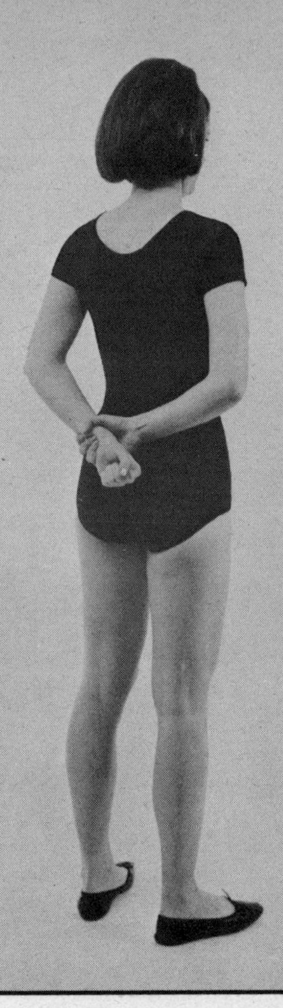

PARADE REST

Position: Stand erect. Place arms behind small of back, grasping left wrist with right hand. Keep chest high, shoulders back.

Contraction: Inhale. Press backs of hands forward against small of back as if you were trying to pass your hands right through your body. Increase pressure for 3 seconds. Hold maximum effort for 4 seconds.

Relax and exhale.

This contraction is especially valuable in strengthening shoulders and upper back. It is one of the best corrective exercises for round shoulders.

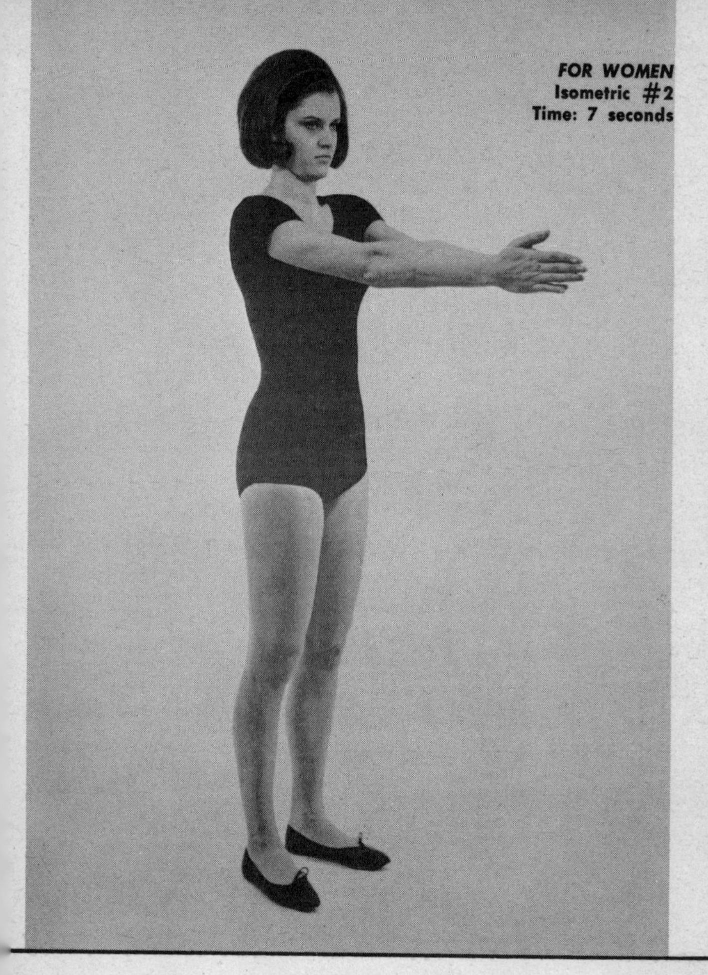

PALM PRESS (ARMS EXTENDED)

Position: Stand erect, arms extended to front, elbows straight, palms together.

Contraction: Inhale. Press palms of hands together, increasing pressure for 3 seconds until maximum effort is reached. Hold maximum effort for 4 seconds.

Relax and exhale.

This contraction firms and strengthens the muscles of the chest beneath the breasts.

FOR WOMEN
Isometric #3
Time: 7 seconds

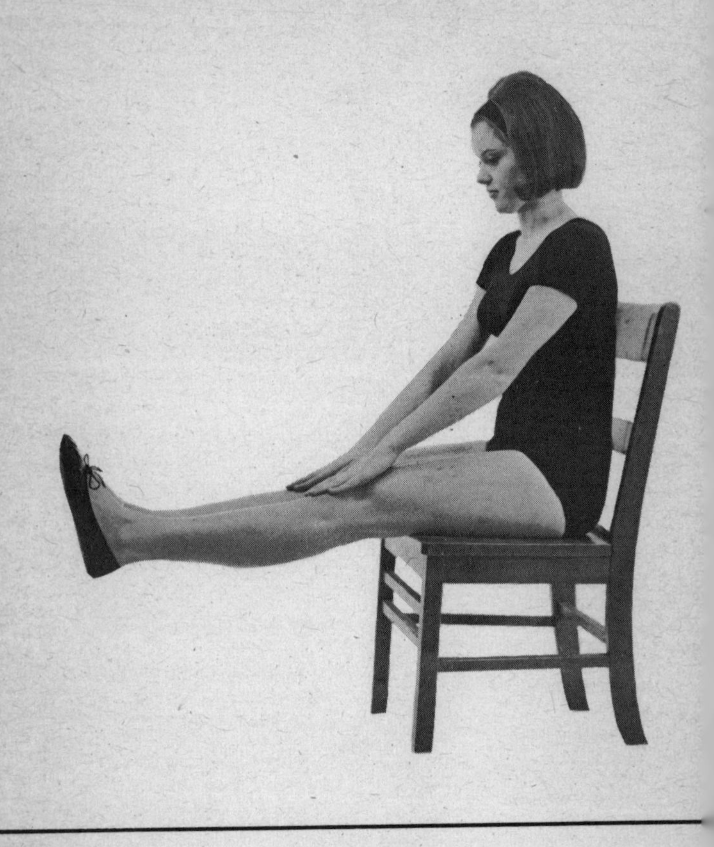

KNEE PRESS

Position: Sit in chair, legs extended, knees straight, heels lifted about a foot off floor. Place palms of hands flat on knees with elbows straight.

Contraction: Inhale. Press down on knees with hands. As you hold legs rigid, increase pressure for 3 seconds. Hold maximum effort for 4 seconds.

Relax and exhale.

This exercise contracts and shortens the muscles that hold in the waistline and is therefore primarily effective around the abdomen.

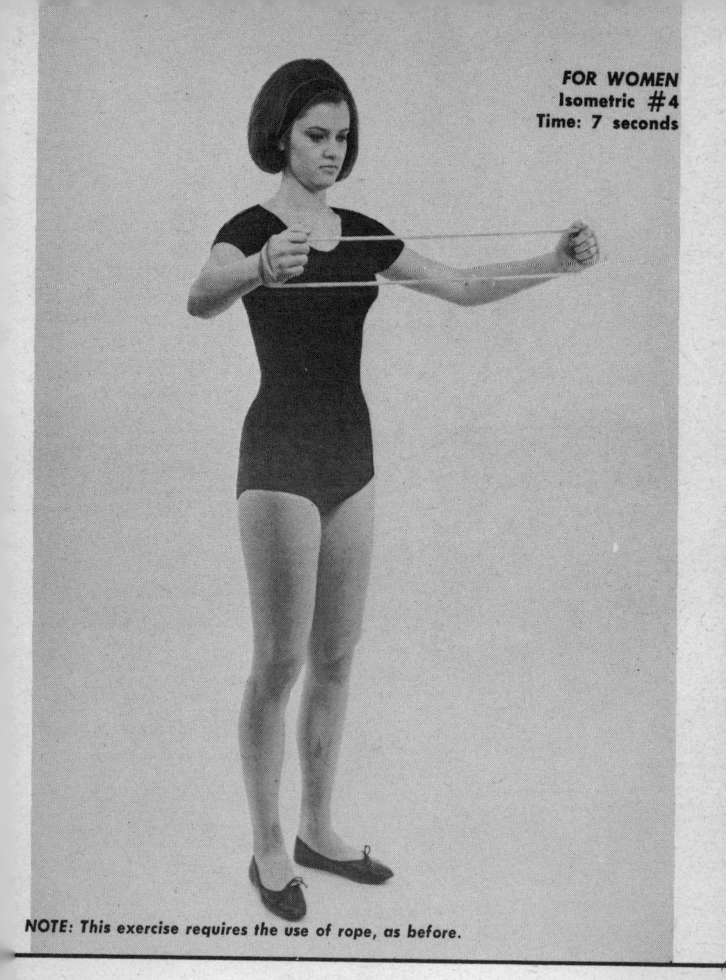

NOTE: This exercise requires the use of rope, as before.

FRONT PULL

Position: Adjust loop so that it is about 2½ to 3 feet in length. Stand erect. Hold loop in front of you about 18 inches from chest, palms inward, elbows slightly bent.

Contraction: Inhale. Attempt to pull loop apart by forcing arms outward. Increase pressure for 3 seconds, hold maximum effort for 4 seconds. Relax and exhale.

This contraction firms up the backs of your arms and strengthens the upper back.

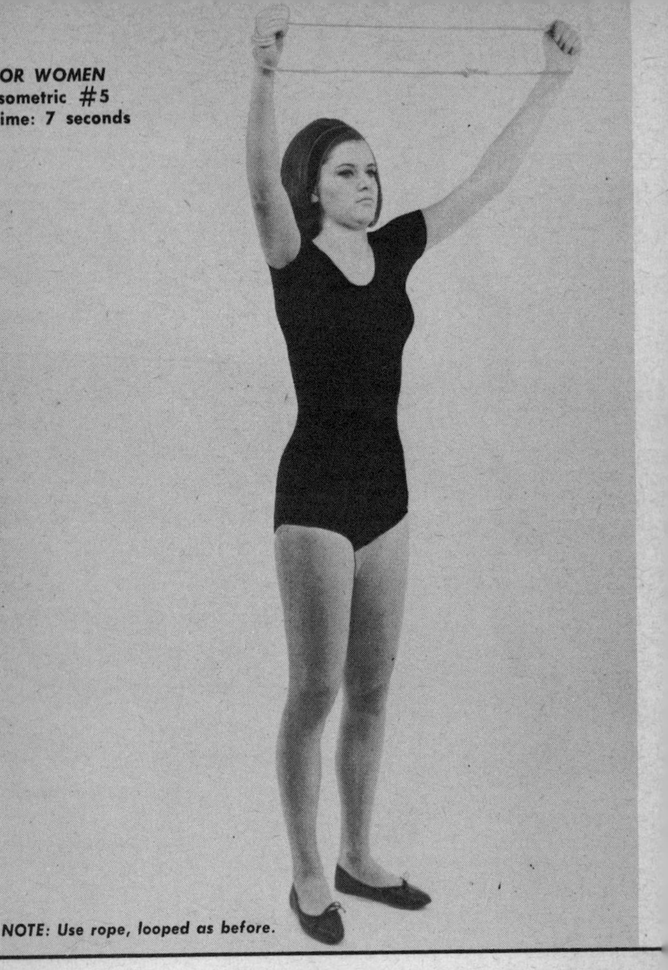

OVERHEAD PULL

Position: Adjust loop so that it is about 2½ to 3 feet in length. Stand erect, hold loop overhead slightly in front of you, palms facing inward.

Contraction: Inhale. Attempt to pull loop apart by forcing arms outward and downward. Increase pressure for 3 seconds, hold maximum effort for 4 seconds.

Relax and exhale.

This contraction strengthens the arms and shoulders and helps to flatten the stomach area.

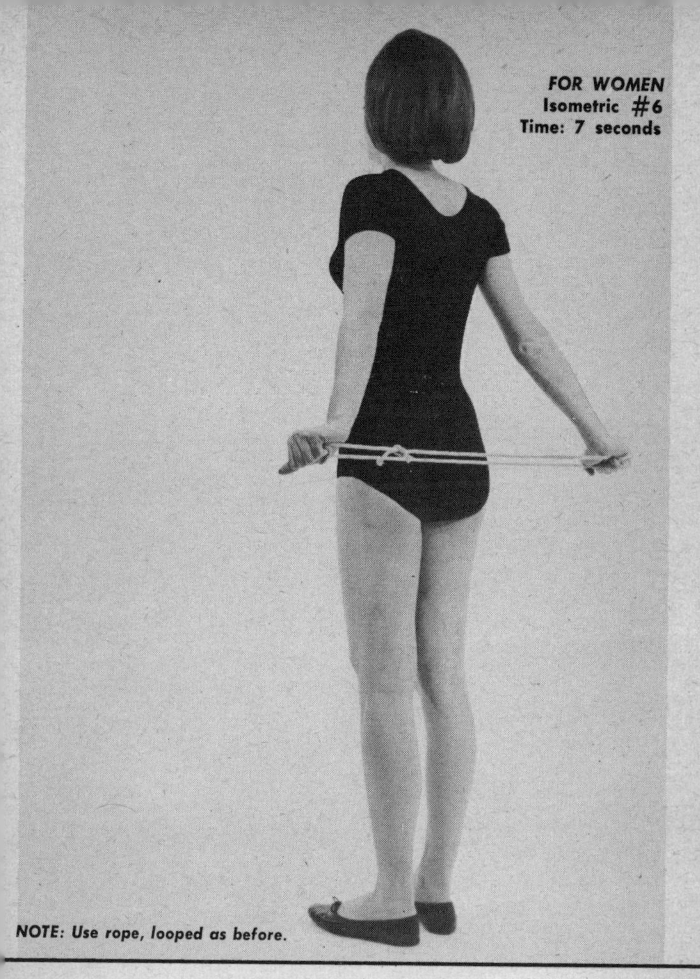

BACK STRETCH AND PULL

Position: Stand erect, chest out. Place loop behind you. Grasp ends of loop with both hands, palms facing down.

Contraction: Inhale. Pull outward and upward on loop, attempting to pull loop apart. Increase effort for 3 seconds until maximum effort is reached. Hold maximum effort for 4 seconds.

Relax and exhale.

This exercise strengthens shoulder and chest areas.

FOR WOMEN
Isometric #7
Time: 7 seconds

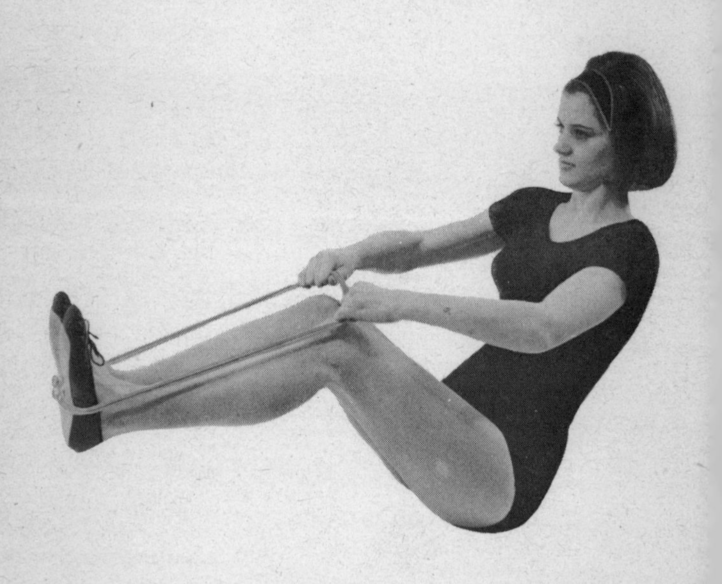

NOTE: Use rope, looped as before.

THIGH PUSH

Position: Sit on floor. Slip loop beneath both feet and grasp ends of loop with both hands. By pulling with arms, lift heels about a foot off floor.

Contraction: Inhale. Attempt to extend legs against counter-pull of arms. Increase pressure for 3 seconds. Hold maximum effort for 4 seconds.

Relax and exhale.

This exercise strengthens and firms muscles of thighs, arms and back.

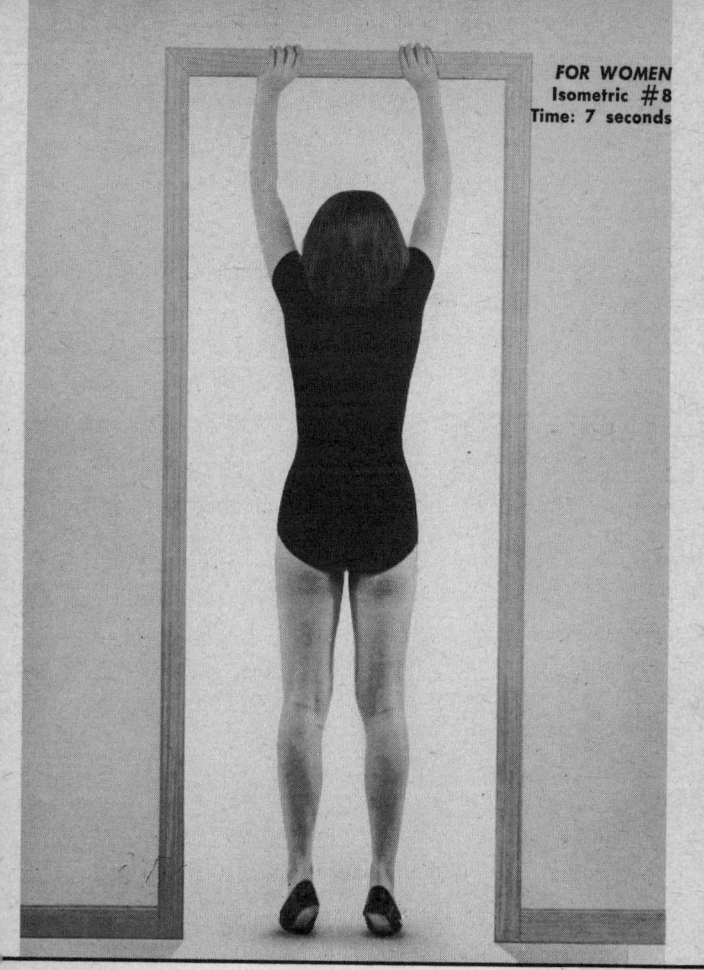

CALF RAISE

Position: Stand in doorway, arms extended overhead with palms flat against top of doorway frame. Raise up on toes so heels are about 3 inches from floor.

Contraction: Inhale. Push top of doorway with arms attempting to force heels to floor. At the same time push back with toes keeping heels up. Increase pressure for 3 seconds. Hold maximum effort for 4 seconds. Relax and exhale.

This exercise is one of the few that build muscle in the calf. If you feel that your calves are developed as much as they should be, do this exercise with the feet flat on the floor thereby using and developing only the muscles of the arms.

FACIAL CONDITIONING EXERCISES
REJUVENATION THROUGH ISOMETRICS

The thirty or so muscles that are responsible for facial movements like chewing, blushing, yawning, etc., have another important function: they form *expressions*. And facial expressions are the calling card we present to people around us.

With the advent of middle age, the muscles of the face often lose their tone and begin to sag. Much of the muscle, too, has been replaced by fatty tissue and the impression of age becomes apparent.

Since facial muscles are composed of the same striated fibers as other voluntary muscles of the body, they respond just as rapidly and just as effectively to the isometric-contraction technique. It has been scientifically demonstrated that isometrics can improve muscle tone and restore firmness to sagging muscles.

So, for a trimmer, more youthful facial appearance, the following isometric contractions should be performed *twice daily*. Effective results should be obtained in just two weeks. Notice that you will not be using the isometric breathing technique (increasing effort *up to* maximum) since the contraction of these small muscles causes no strain whatever on the body.

Isometric
Time: 10 seconds

Isometric #1. Holding your mouth open as wide as possible, simultaneously attempt to purse your lips as though to whistle. Exert maximum effort for 10 seconds without closing mouth.

Isometric #2. With your thumb and forefinger inside your mouth, press them against the insides of both cheeks. With fingers, attempt to force cheeks apart and at the same time try to force the thumb and forefinger together. Exert maximum effort for 10 seconds.

Isometric #3. Hold your forefinger about 3 inches away from your lips. Try to touch your finger with your lips *without moving your head forward.* Hold maximum effort for 10 seconds.

Isometric #4. Half smile—using the *left side* of your mouth only—while you close your *right* eye as tightly as possible. Hold maximum effort for 10 seconds.

Isometric #5. Smile with the *right side* of your mouth and simultaneously close your *left* eye as tightly as you can. Hold maximum effort for 10 seconds.

PART III

HOW TO IMPROVE YOUR SPORTS-PERFORMANCE WITH ISOMETRIC CONTRACTIONS

Isometric-contraction techniques, when applied to sports, can be of great value. Marked improvement in athletic performance is evident when these techniques have been made part of the athlete's training program. This is true even when the athlete has been training to the limit of his capacity with conventional methods. With the introduction of isometrics into his program, the athlete's level of performance invariably goes up.

Bob Hoffman, Olympic coach and a leading exponent of body building, states: "Functional isometric contraction is especially applicable to the training for many sports. It is the best and fastest way to build strength, which is the most important characteristic of an athlete regardless of what sport he practices."

National champion weightlifters, finding their lifting capabilities levelled off while using conventional training methods, soon discovered a great increase in that lifting capacity when isometrics were used.

Golfer Gary Player adopted the system to strengthen the back, forearm and leg muscles which help him to drive a longer ball.

In track and field sports, such National Champions as discus-thrower Jay Sylvester, sprinter Frank Budd, and high-jumper Bob Avant attribute a large measure of their successful performances to the inclusion of contraction exercises in their training programs.

One aspect of isometrics is especially applicable to sports: The force of a specific movement can be increased *exactly at the point where it is most needed.* For example, when a football player is kicking, he must exert *maximum force* at the point when his foot comes in contact with the ball. The isometric contraction for this movement, then, is applied with the foot and leg in exactly that position.

Individuals interested in improving their sports-performance through isometric contractions must go about this in two ways: Initially, they should perform those contractions that first build overall body strength. The isometric contractions described in the Secondary Level will increase body strength no matter how strong you are to start with.

Secondly, the athlete should perform, daily, those isometric contractions that apply to his particular sport.

The isometric contractions described in the following section, then, will increase strength and performance. They can be done in less than one minute a day for each sport, and are as effective for teenagers and women as they are for the strongest athlete.

To obtain maximum benefit, the athlete must perform each contraction *for the full ten seconds,* allowing the previously mentioned *overload principle* to come into play.

For those taking the total-fitness program, the isometrics designed to improve your sports-performance should follow the warm-up period at each Level.

And remember: In isometric contractions *there is no movement.*

These exercises are to be done *ONLY ONCE.*

GOLF

In golf the application of the isometric technique aids those who wish to hit a longer ball. The following exercises, if done daily, will strengthen both you and your game. All the equipment you'll need are a broomstick and a piece of rope or clothesline, as before.

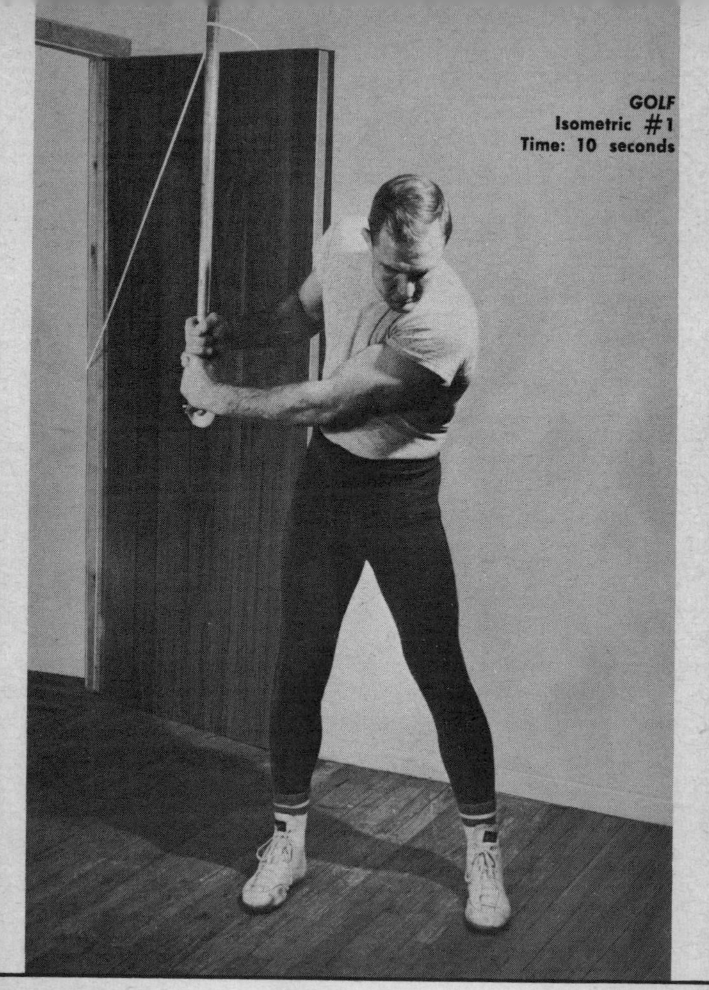

SWING START

Position: Tie an 8-foot section of clothesline or rope to the end of a stick. Attach the rope's other end to a fixed object (a door knob, for instance). Hold the stick with your regular grip and assume a stance where the stick is in the position of the start of your down swing. Adjust yourself so that the rope becomes taut and you cannot move the stick.

Contraction: Inhale. Pull downward with your arms holding wrists rigid, increase effort for 4 seconds. Hold maximum effort for 6 seconds.

Relax and exhale.

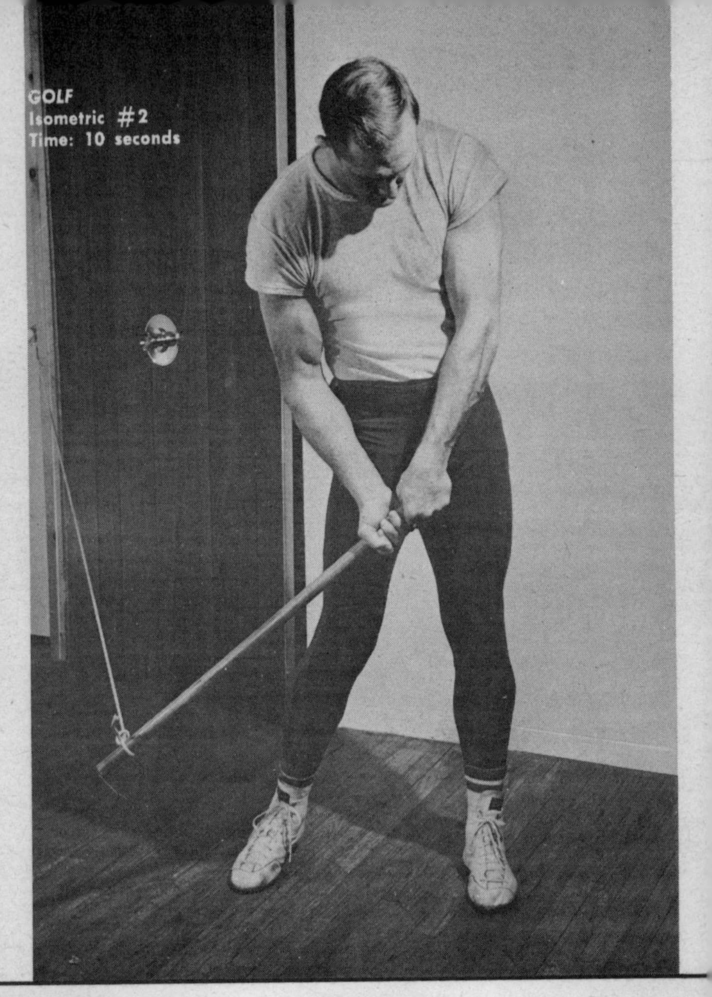

MIDSWING

Position: Bring stick to mid-swing position and draw rope taut so that you cannot continue motion.

Contraction: Inhale. Press against rope with stick, increasing pressure for 4 seconds. Hold maximum for 6 seconds. Relax and exhale.

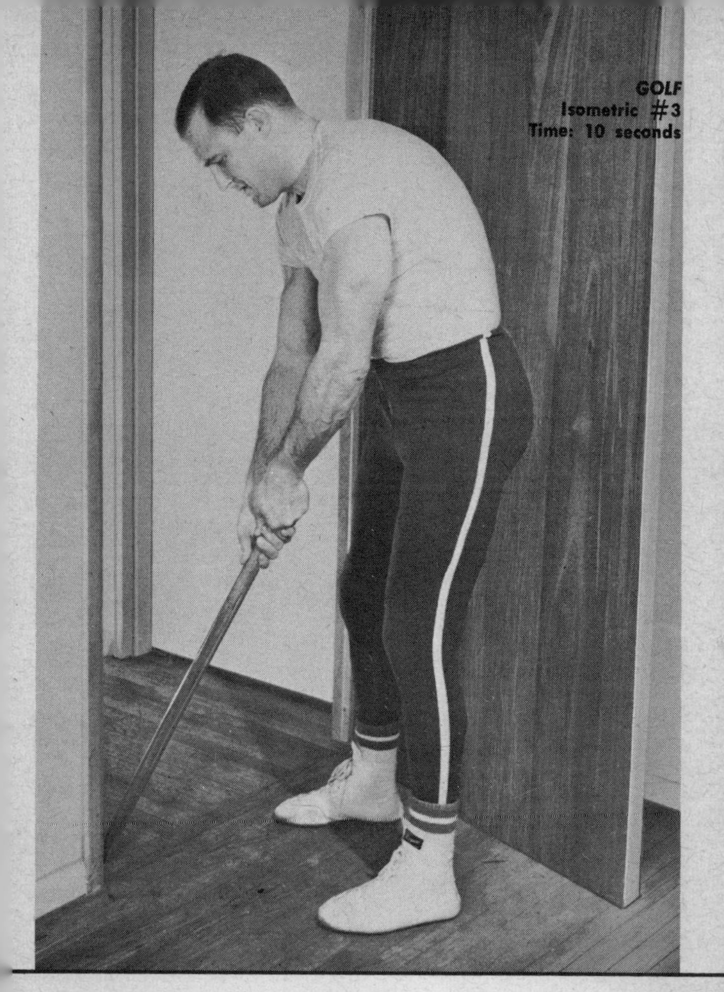

IMPACT

Position: Grasp end of a broomstick cut to the length of your wood or driving iron. Use your regular golfing grip. Arrange your position against the side of a doorway or other immovable obstacle so that the end of the stick is touching the side of the doorway, at exactly the same point that you would normally strike a teed-up ball. (The stick is touching the wall so that there is no movement.)

Contraction: Inhale. Apply pressure to the wall with the stick while you are in the driving stance. Increase pressure for 4 seconds until you have reached your maximum effort. Hold maximum effort for 6 seconds. Relax and exhale.

(NOTE: Do not bend your wrists when applying pressure.)

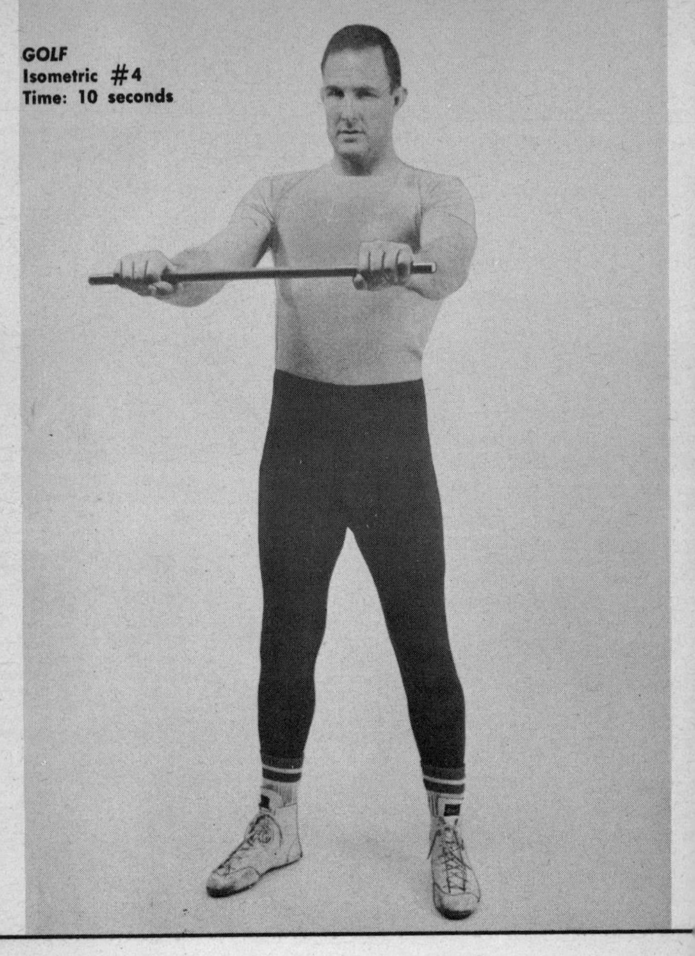

WRIST AND FOREARM BUILDER (#1)

Position: Palms down, grasp broomstick at both ends. Hold stick in front of chest about 10 inches.

Contraction: Inhale. Keeping wrists firm, force elbows down as though to snap stick in two. *Do not move arms.* Pressure will be felt in the wrists, and should be increased for 4 seconds. Hold maximum effort for 6 seconds.

Relax and exhale.

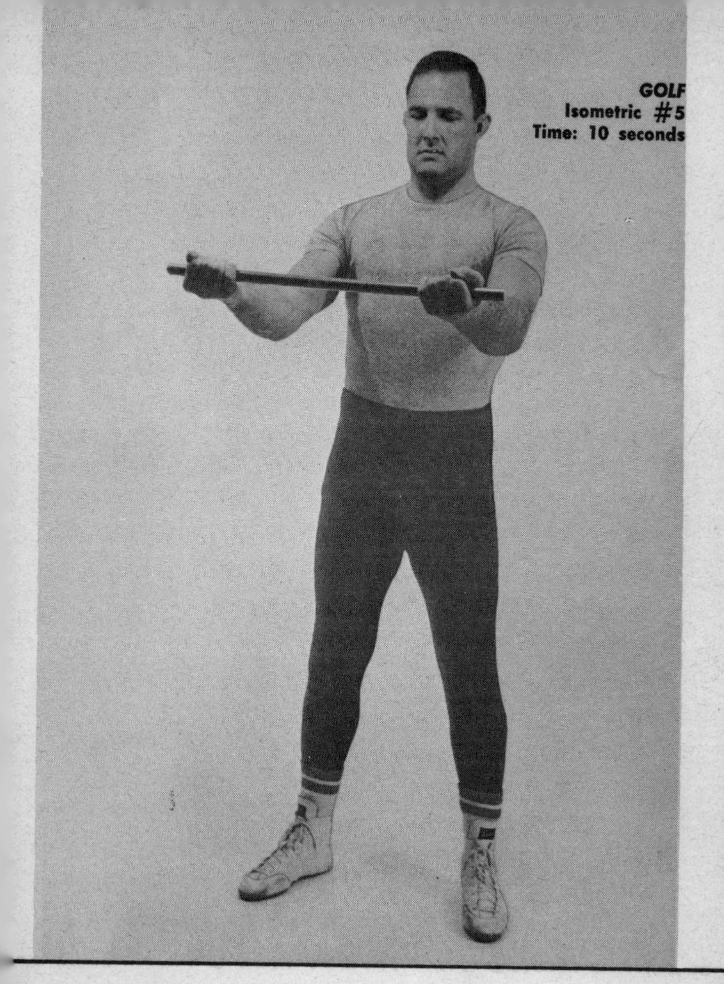

WRIST AND FOREARM BUILDER (#2)

Position: Same as in preceding exercise except palms are held *facing upward.*

Contraction: Inhale. Exert pressure upward for 4 seconds. Hold maximum effort for 6 seconds.

Relax and exhale.

TENNIS

Isometric contractions in relation to tennis concentrate on two major areas: the player's arms and legs.

In this game, especially in singles, the demands on the player are enormous. Thus total fitness is especially important. *People over 40 are advised to play only doubles, and then only if physically on a par with what is expected for the Secondary Level of the Total-Fitness Plan.*

To improve your game, perform the following isometric contractions daily. If you do not play tennis regularly, use the following in conjunction with your level of the isometric-isotonic Total-Fitness Plan, in which case these exercises should be done following the warm-up period of your particular level.

In performing these contractions, use an old racket or broomstick cut to the length of a tennis racket.

These exercises are to be done *ONLY ONCE.*

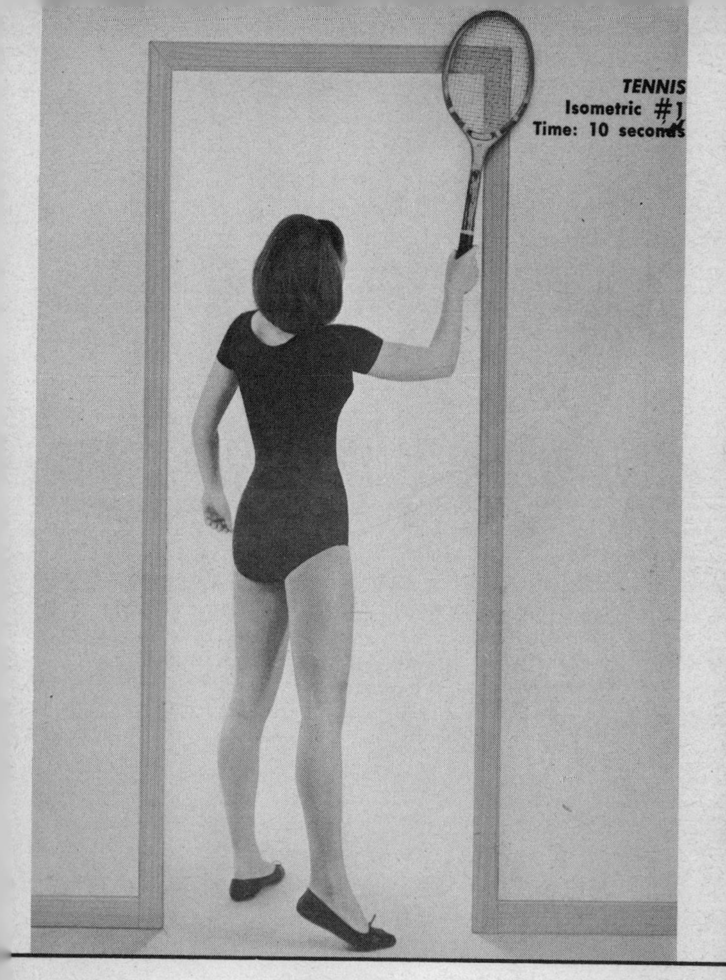

THE SERVE

Position: Stand in a doorway with the racket or stick in your playing hand, regular grip. Place the face of the racket or stick against the top of the doorway while you assume the stance that you would normally take at the top of your serve.

Contraction: Inhale. Holding wrist firm, press racket or stick against top of doorway, increasing pressure for 4 seconds until maximum effort is reached. Hold maximum effort for 6 seconds. Relax and exhale.

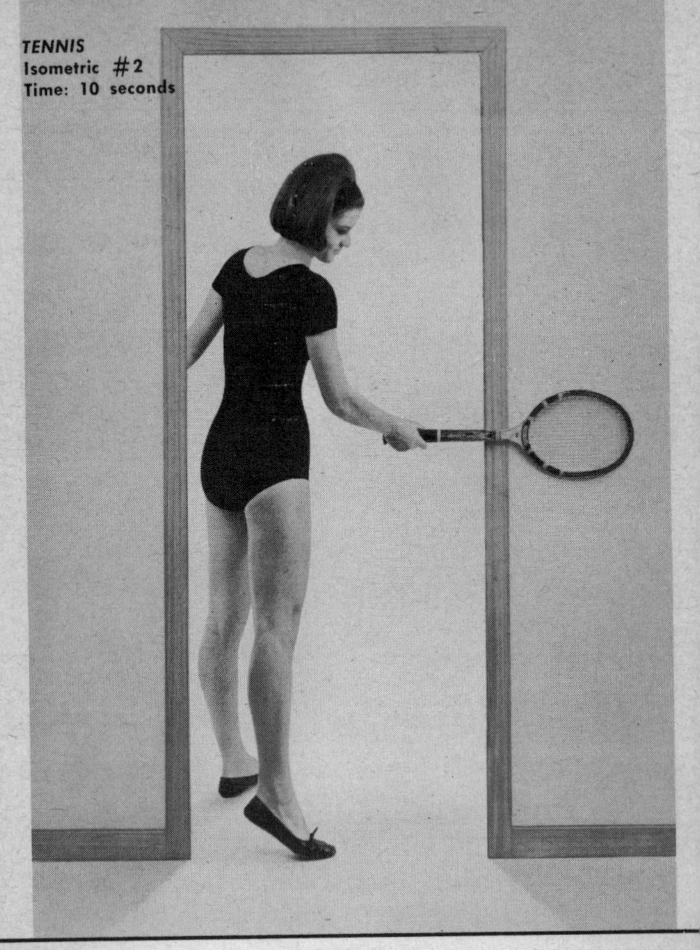

FOREHAND SWING

Position: Stand in doorway assuming stance of forehand swing. Place face of racket against side of doorway at point where your racket would normally come in contact with the ball in a forehand swing.

Contraction: Inhale. Holding wrist firm, press racket against side of doorway, using shoulder and arm. Increase pressure for 4 seconds until you reach your maximum effort. Hold maximum effort for 6 seconds. Relax and exhale.

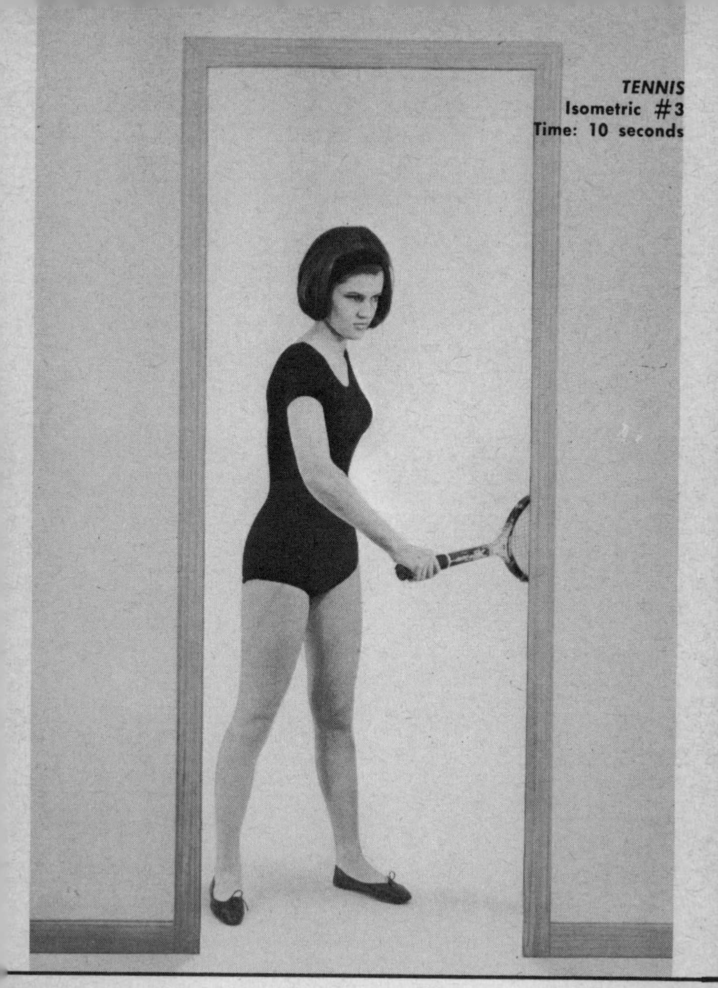

BACKHAND SWING

Position: Stand in doorway, assuming backhand-swing stance in exactly the same position as in the instant that the racket would come in contact with the ball. At this point the racket should be in contact with, and pressing against, the side of the doorway's frame.

Contraction: Inhale. Holding wrist firm, press racket against side of doorway. Increase pressure for 4 seconds until maximum effort is reached. Hold maximum effort for 6 seconds.

Relax and exhale.

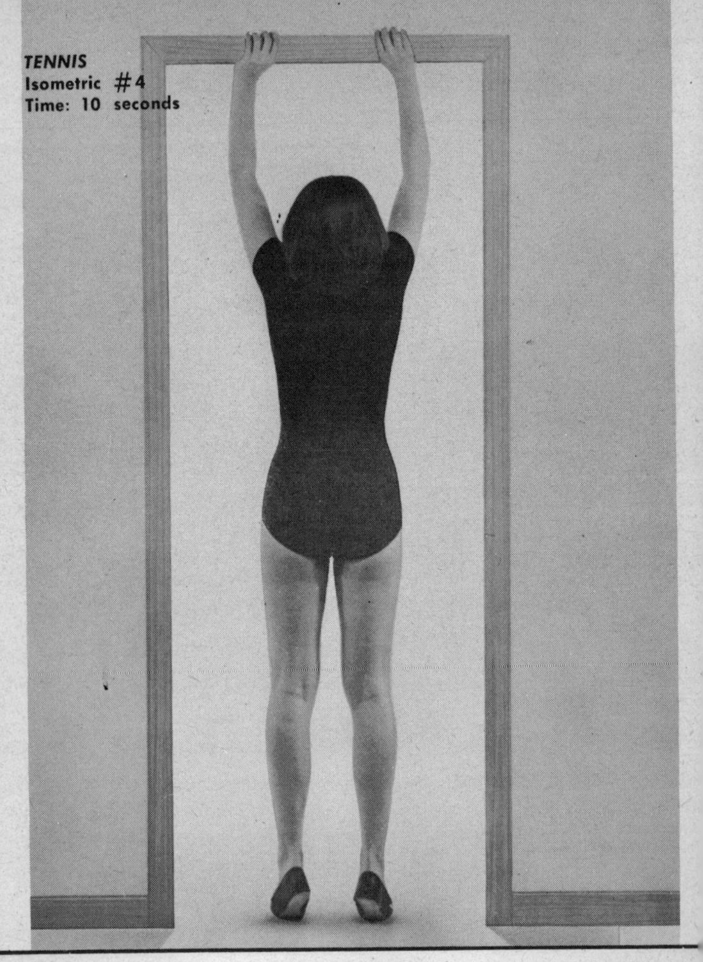

TOE RAISER

Position: Stand erect in doorway. Raise arms, placing hands against top of doorway. If you cannot reach top of doorway, stand on books or other firm base. Now rise up halfway on toes.

Contraction: Inhale. Push *up* against top of doorway with arms, attempting to force heels down to the floor. Simultaneously, push up with calves of legs so heels are prevented from going down. Increase pressure for 4 seconds. Hold maximum effort for 6 seconds.

Relax and exhale.

***NOTE:** Perform this exercise again immediately. This second time, the start position is up on your toes as high as you can go.*

SWIMMING

Speed swimming requires strength in the whiplash action of the leg kick, and in the pull and recovery of the arms. The action varies, however, in the different strokes, and these exercises can be modified for use in the particular stroke you are trying to perfect.

For all-around, or medley, swimmers, all the exercises should be done.

Others need only be concerned with the few exercises that pertain to a stroke of particular interest to them.

The exercises described should be executed just as decribed by swimmers who are in training, who should do them at least six times each, at various times throughout the day.

SWIMMING
Isometric #1
Time: 10 seconds

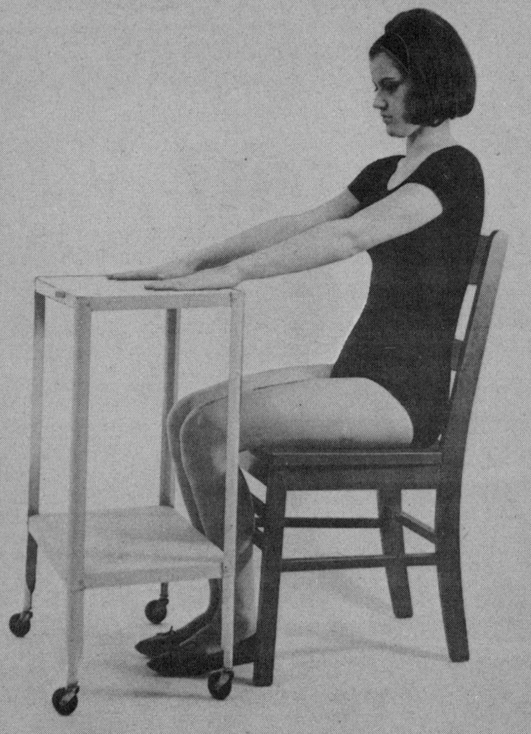

CRAWL AND BUTTERFLY ARM-ACTION (ENTRY)

Position: Sit at a table, arms extended in front of you, palms down flat on table.

Contraction: Inhale. Press down on table attempting to lift yourself out of your seat with the downward pressure of your arms. Increase pressure for 4 seconds. Hold maximum effort for 6 seconds. Relax and exhale.

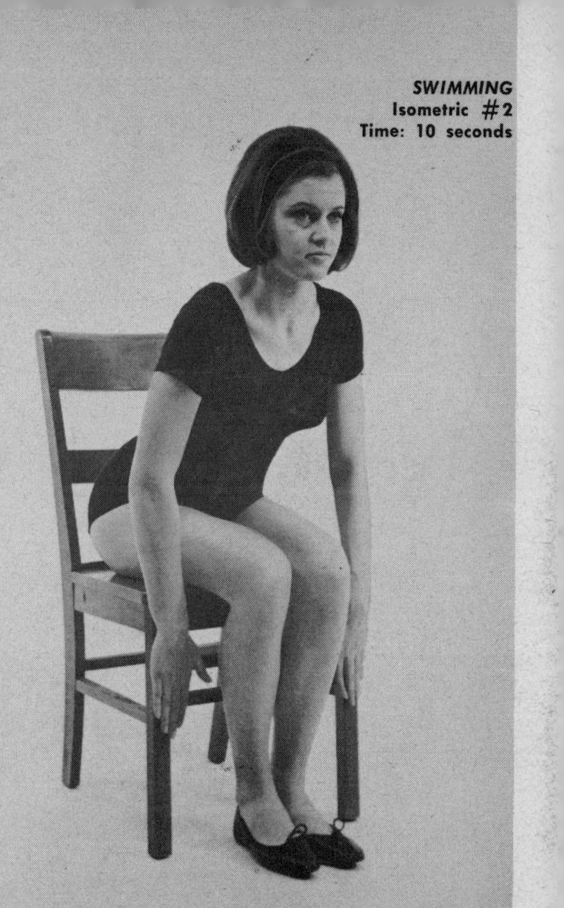

CRAWL AND BUTTERFLY ARM-ACTION (RECOVERY)

Position: Sit erect in chair, legs together, arms extended down sides of chair legs. Place palms against front of chair seat on each side.

Contraction: Inhale. Press palms of hands against each side of seat increasing pressure for 4 seconds. Hold maximum effort for 6 seconds. Relax and exhale.

SWIMMING
Isometric #3
Time: 10 seconds

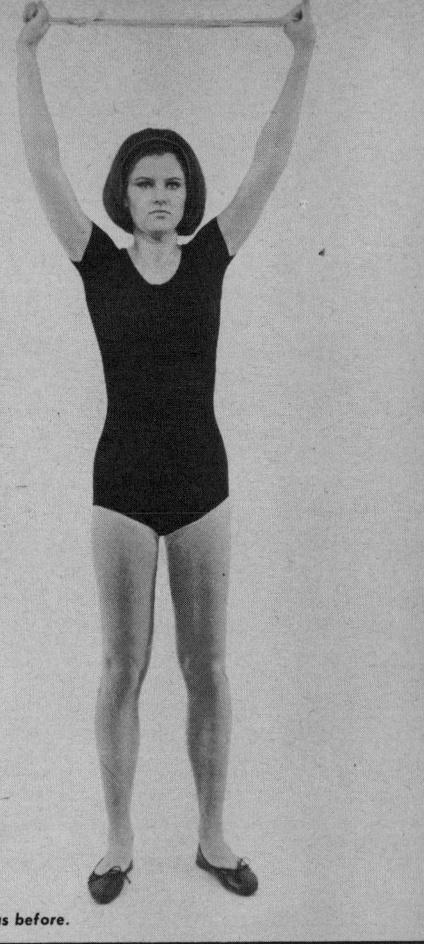

NOTE: Use looped rope, as before.

BACK STROKE ARM-ACTION

Position: Stand or sit erect. Adjust loop so that arms are in relatively same position as when they enter the water. Place both arms over head grasping ends of loop with palms outward.

Contraction: Inhale. Force arms against loop outward and downward. Increase pressure for 4 seconds. Hold maximum effort for 6 seconds. Relax and exhale.

Time: 10 seconds

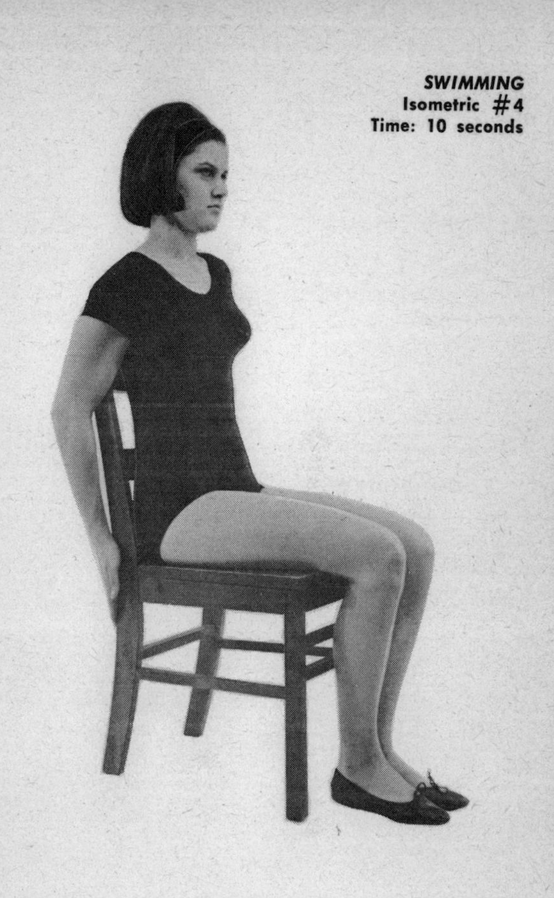

BACK STROKE ARM-ACTION (RECOVERY)

Position: Sit erect in chair. Elbows straight, place palms of hands, one on each side, against back legs of chair.

Contraction: Inhale. Force arms forward, pressing palms of hands against back legs of chair. Increase pressure for 4 seconds. Hold maximum effort for 6 seconds. Relax and exhale.

SWIMMING
Isometric #5
Time: 10 seconds

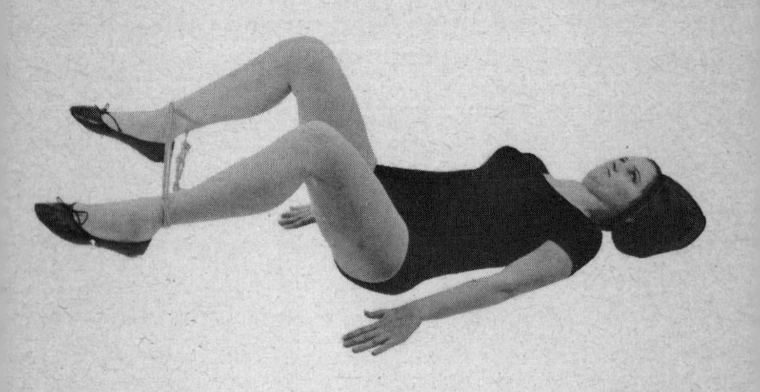

NOTE: Use looped rope, as before.

BREAST STROKE LEG-ACTION

Position: Adjust loop to about 2 feet in length. Lay on back and slip loop on, just above ankles. Bend knees to position at start of kick.

Contraction: Inhale. Force legs apart against loop, increasing pressure for 4 seconds. Hold maximum effort for 6 seconds. Relax and exhale.

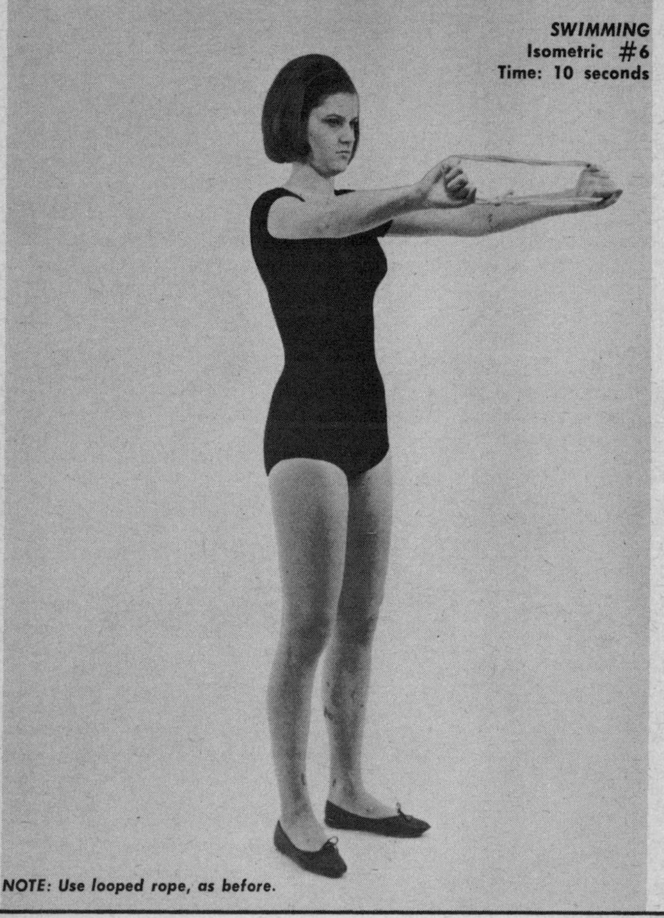

BREAST STROKE ARM-ACTION

Position: Adjust loop to 30 inches or to a length that conforms to that of the start of your pull. Hold loop in front of you at arm's length, hands inside, palms facing outward, thumbs pointing to floor.

Contraction: Inhale. Force arms outward against loop, increasing pressure for 4 seconds. Hold maximum effort for 6 seconds. Relax and exhale.

Isometric #7
Time: 10 seconds

CRAWL AND BACK STROKE LEG-ACTION

***NOTE:** Use looped rope, as before.*

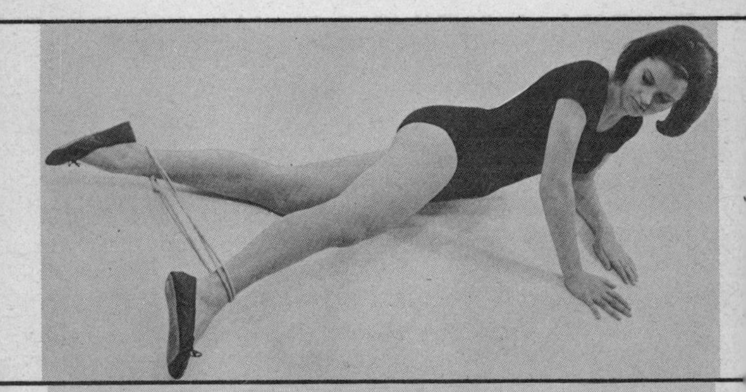

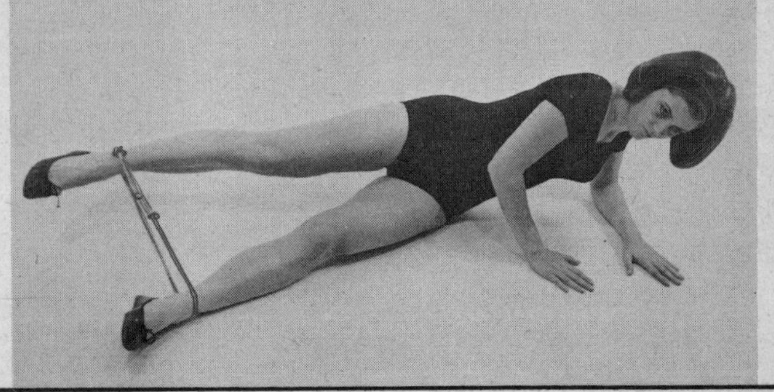

Position: Adjust loop to slip about both ankles so that feet, when held in a stride position, are about 13 inches apart. Lay on floor or bench on either your left or right side, with loop placed around both ankles.

Contraction: Inhale. With knees slightly bent, force right leg forward, left leg backward against loop, increasing pressure for 4 seconds until maximum effort is reached. Hold maximum effort for 6 seconds. Relax and exhale.

Repeat this contraction placing your left leg forward and your right leg back.

SKIING

When applied to skiing, the benefit of isometric contractions in the skier's training program is two-fold: First, by making the skier stronger he can perform movements more confidently and thus more skillfully. Secondly, the body's joints, tendons and ligaments, strengthened by these exercises, are less prone to injury.

In this sport, where the seasonal lay-off period is long, and sudden strains are the rule rather than the exception, isometrics are a must.

These isometrics for skiers should be started about five weeks before the first outing, and may also be used as a warm-up before actually starting a run.

It is strongly recommended that the Total-Fitness Plan be made an integral part of your pre-season training schedule.

These exercises are to be done *ONLY ONCE.*

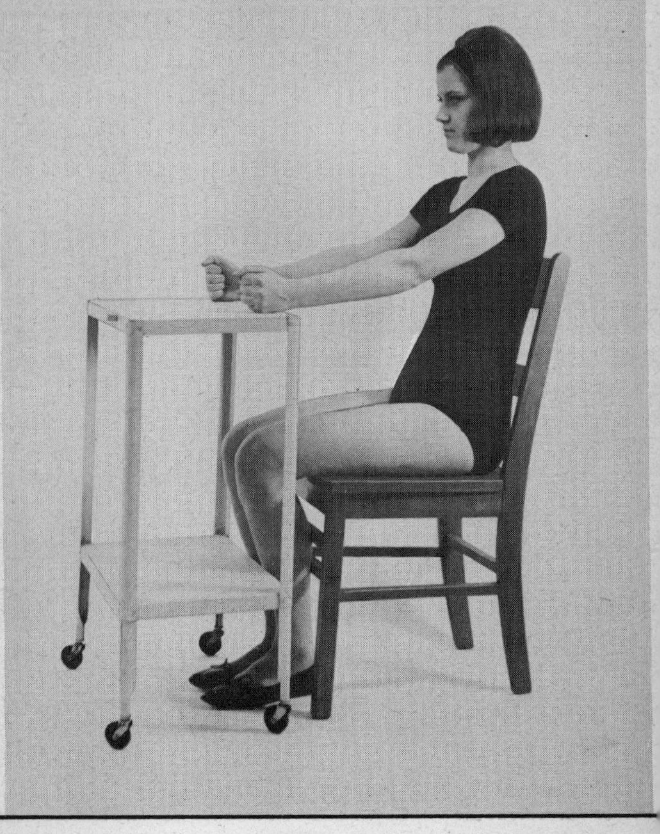

ARM PRESS

Position: Sit at table with arms extended, fists clenched and resting on table, thumbs up.

Contraction: Inhale. Attempt to lift yourself up from chair by pressing down on table with fists. Increase pressure for 4 seconds. Hold maximum effort for 6 seconds. Relax and exhale.

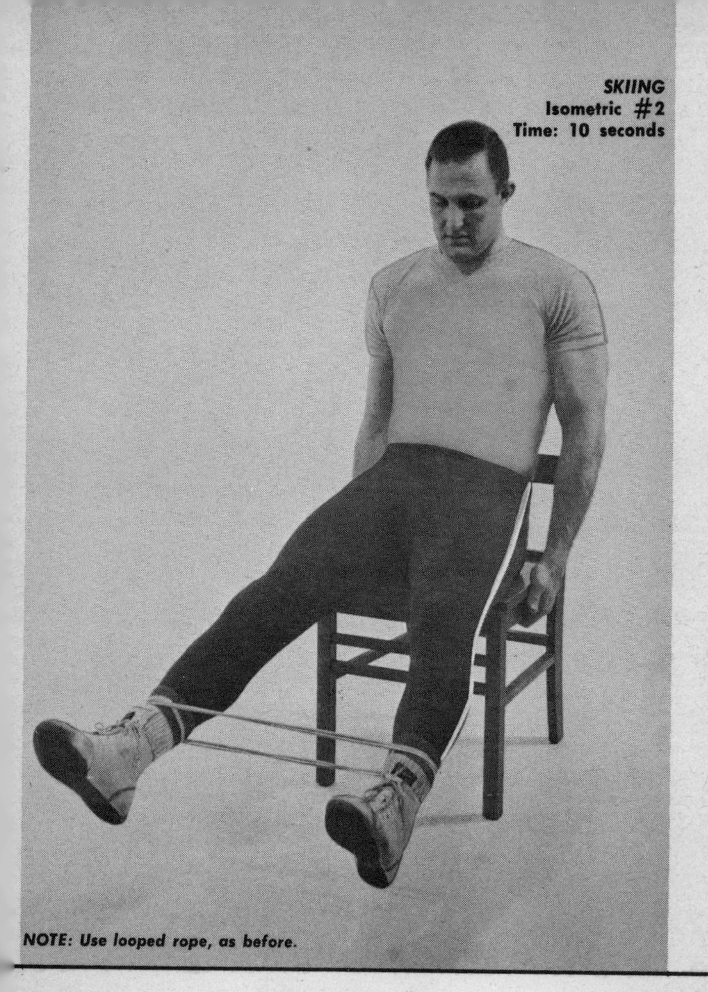

LEG ABDUCTOR

Position: Adjust loop to 24 inches in length. Sit in chair with legs extended, heels about a foot off the floor. Place loop around both ankles.

Contraction: Inhale. Force legs outward and apart against loop. Increase pressure for 4 seconds. Hold maximum effort for 6 seconds. Relax and exhale.

LEG EXTENSOR

NOTE: Use looped rope, as before.

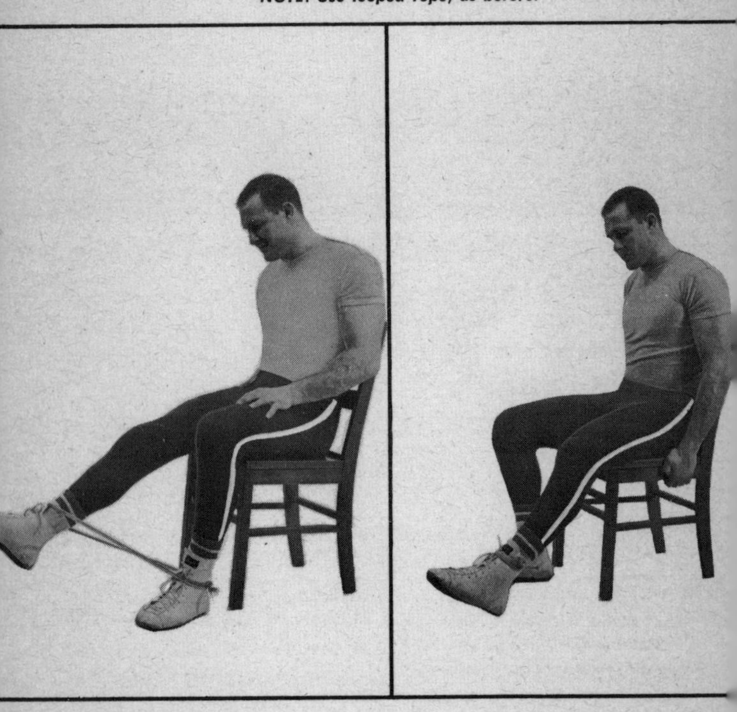

Position: Sit on chair. Place loop around ankles.

Contraction: Inhale. Force right leg forward keeping left foot flat on the floor. Increase effort for 4 seconds. Hold maximum effort for 6 seconds. Relax and exhale. Repeat action with left leg.

KNEE-PRESS (INTERIOR)

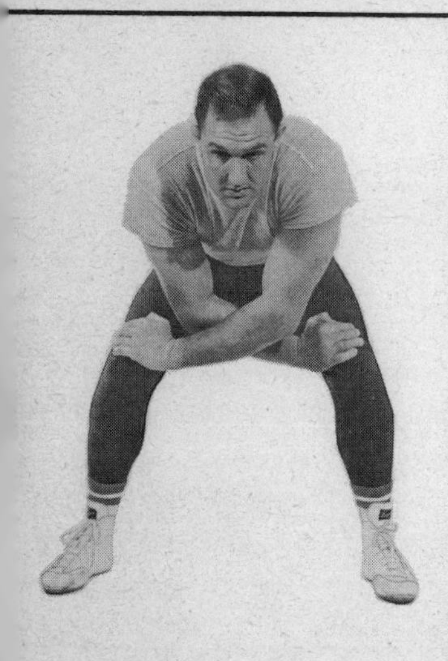

Position: Semi-squat forward, cross arms and place palms of hands against *insides* of opposite knees.

Contraction: Inhale. Press palms outward against insides of knees and simultaneously try to force knees together. Increase effort for 4 seconds until maximum effort is reached. Hold maximum effort for 6 seconds.

Relax and exhale.

KNEE PRESS (EXTERIOR)

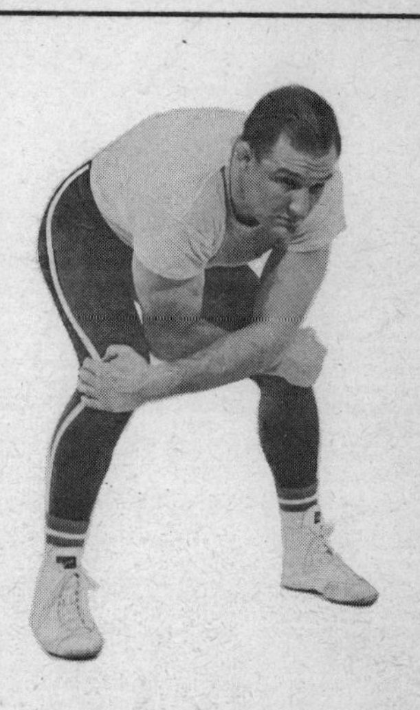

Position: Semi-squat forward. Cross arms and grasp outside of opposite knees.

Contraction: Inhale. Attempt to pull knees together with hands, at the same time force knees apart with legs. Increase effort for 4 seconds and hold maximum effort for 6 seconds.

Relax and exhale.

ISOMETRIC CONTRACTIONS FOR TEAM SPORTS

Isometric contractions develop strength and explosiveness in the power movements required in team sports. Professional, amateur and college stars now include this form of training in all their workouts.

In the big three team sports, baseball, basketball, and football, the large muscles of the legs, back, and hips have terrific demands made on them. These are the areas where isometrics can show spectacular results.

In addition to the series of ten isometric contractions described previously in the Secondary and Peak Levels of the Total-Fitness Plan, the following exercises should be included. They may be done *only once.*

TEAM SPORTS
Isometric #1
Time: 10 seconds

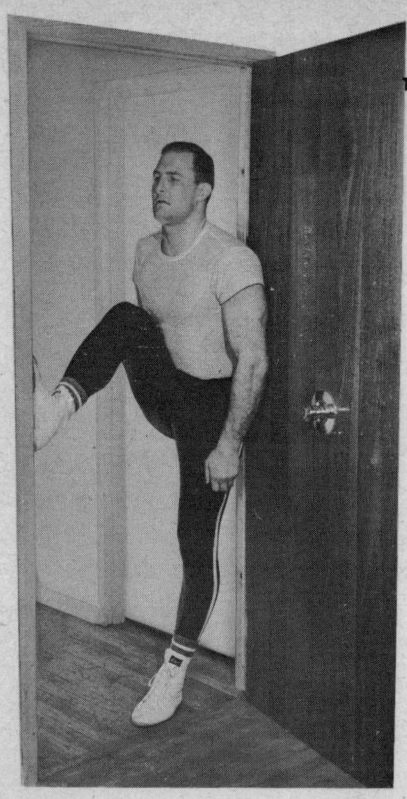

This exercise will develop tremendous power in the thighs and is indicated for all the major team sports.

In this exercise, be sure to select a doorway strong enough to withstand the pressure you will be exerting against it.

QUADRICEPS-PUSH

Position: Stand in doorway with back against one side of frame. Raise one leg and place foot flat against opposite frame at hip height.

Contraction: Inhale. Attempt to straighten leg by pushing against side of doorway. Increase pressure for 4 seconds at which time you should be exerting maximum effort. Hold maximum effort for 6 seconds. Relax and exhale.

Repeat this contraction, alternating with each leg.

TEAM SPORTS
Isometric #2
Time: 10 seconds

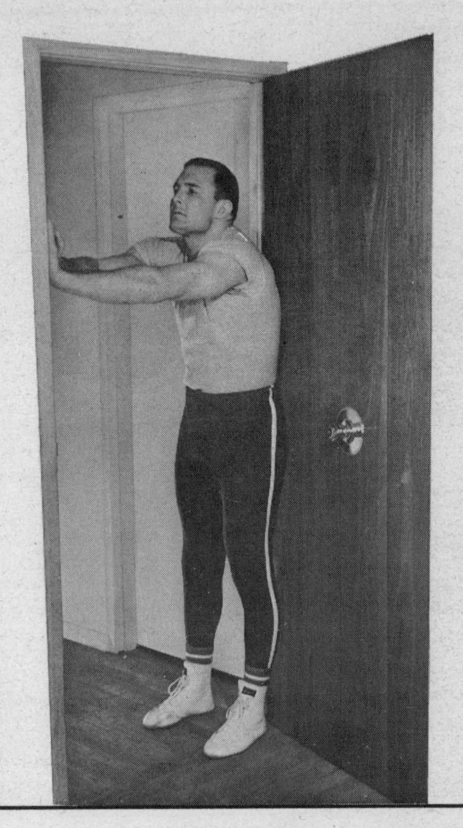

FRONT PRESS

Position: Stand in doorway with back against one side of frame. Extend both arms so that palms of hands are flat against opposite frame.

Contraction: Inhale. Push with arms against frame as back presses against opposite side of doorway. Increase pressure for 4 seconds. Hold maximum effort for 6 seconds. Relax and exhale.

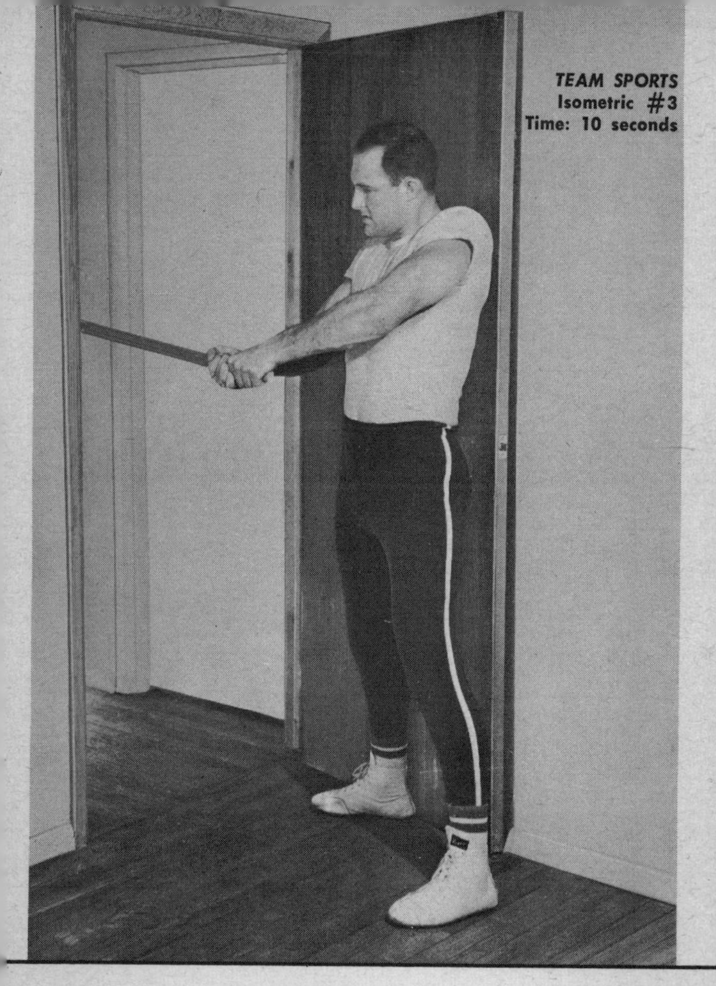

TEAM SPORTS
Isometric #3
Time: 10 seconds

BATTER'S SWING

Position: Assume batting stance near doorway. Hold stick as you would a baseball bat, placing it against side of doorway at height that you would normally strike a baseball.

Contraction: Inhale. Press stick against doorway, wrists firm, increasing pressure for 4 seconds. Hold maximum effort for 6 seconds. Relax and exhale.

This contraction can also help increase the power of your tennis side-arm swing.

NOTE: This exercise requires the use of a broomstick.

IN CONCLUSION . . .

The objective of this book has been to help you add to your capacity for living a healthier, more vigorous, and, consequently, a happier life. It has been demonstrated that regular exercise, keyed to the level of individual capacity, is an integral factor in reaching this objective. Total fitness, however, requires a logical pattern that should include the following:

●

AVOID TENSIONS. Middle-aged people have a tendency to worry more than younger people (perhaps they have more to worry about!) But fretting isn't going to help you live a well-balanced life. Peace of mind is a tall order, but a vital one.

●

GET ADEQUATE REST. The amount of sleep you need depends on you as an individual and therefore varies from person to person. In addition to getting enough sleep, though, try to allow time for rest periods during the day. A short rest can go a long way to alleviate tension.

●

RELAX AFTER MEALS. If possible, this short rest after eating should be a daily habit. And after exercising, you should always allow for a cooling-off period.

●

OBSERVE THE RULES OF PERSONAL HYGIENE. In addition to being more attractive, cleanliness supplies you with one of the essentials to health and well-being.

●

OBSERVE THE RULES OF GOOD NUTRITION. In the final analysis, you are what you eat. Simple, wholesome foods are available to most of us throughout the year and are usually less expensive than spicy, over-rich prepared meats and pastries. Vitamin supplements might also be healthful, particularly during the winter months.

●

EXERCISE REGULARLY. Exercise will help you feel younger, but must not be overdone, particularly by people over forty. Ageing may be inexorable, but the best way to live each year is by getting the most out of each year. Exercise can help by supplying the healthy body that makes an important contribution to a full, rich life.